Does this look good on me?

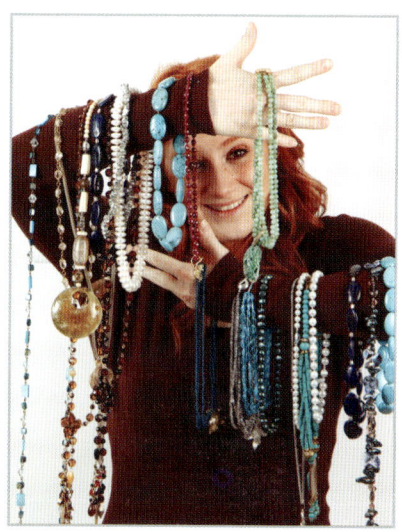

Choose the jewellery to suit your looks,

for an amazing image, always

By Karen Faulkner-Dunkley

THE WORDSMITH PRESS

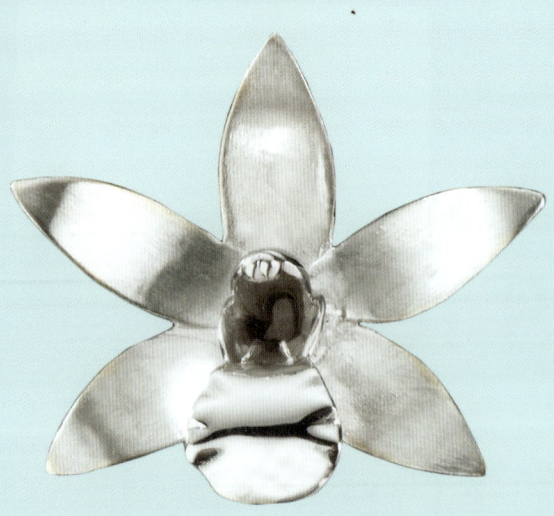

© Copyright Karen Faulkner-Dunkley 2012

Does this Look Good on Me?
Choose the jewellery to suit your looks,
for an amazing image, always

Karen Faulkner-Dunkley

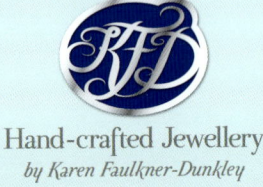

Hand-crafted Jewellery
by Karen Faulkner-Dunkley

Published 2012
The Wordsmith Press
72 Oxford Street
Woodstock
OX20 1TX

THE WORDSMITH PRESS

All rights reserved. Apart from limited use for private study, teaching, research, criticism or review, no part of this publication may be reproduced, stored or transmitted without the prior permission in writing of the copyright owner and publisher of this book.

ISBN 978-0-9560795-1-0

Typeset in Palatino and printed in Great Britain by
LDI Print, New Yatt, Witney OX29 6SZ

Cover and interior design by Clockwork Graphic Design
www.clockworkgraphicdesign.co.uk

Contents

About the Author	5
Introduction	7
Colour Test	9
Face Shape	17
Earrings	27
Necklaces	33
Hand and Wrist Size: bracelets, bangles and rings	41
Colour and Jewellery	47
Personality	65
Occasions	77
Holiday Jewellery	81
About the Designers	89
Putting it all Together	105
Acknowledgements	106

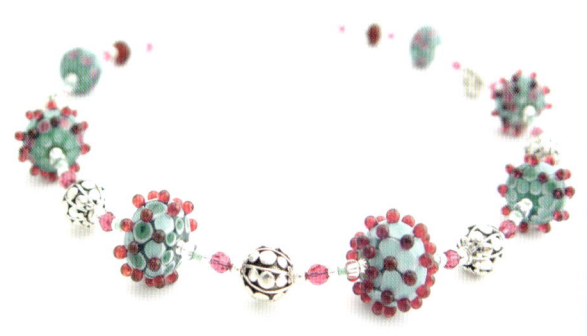

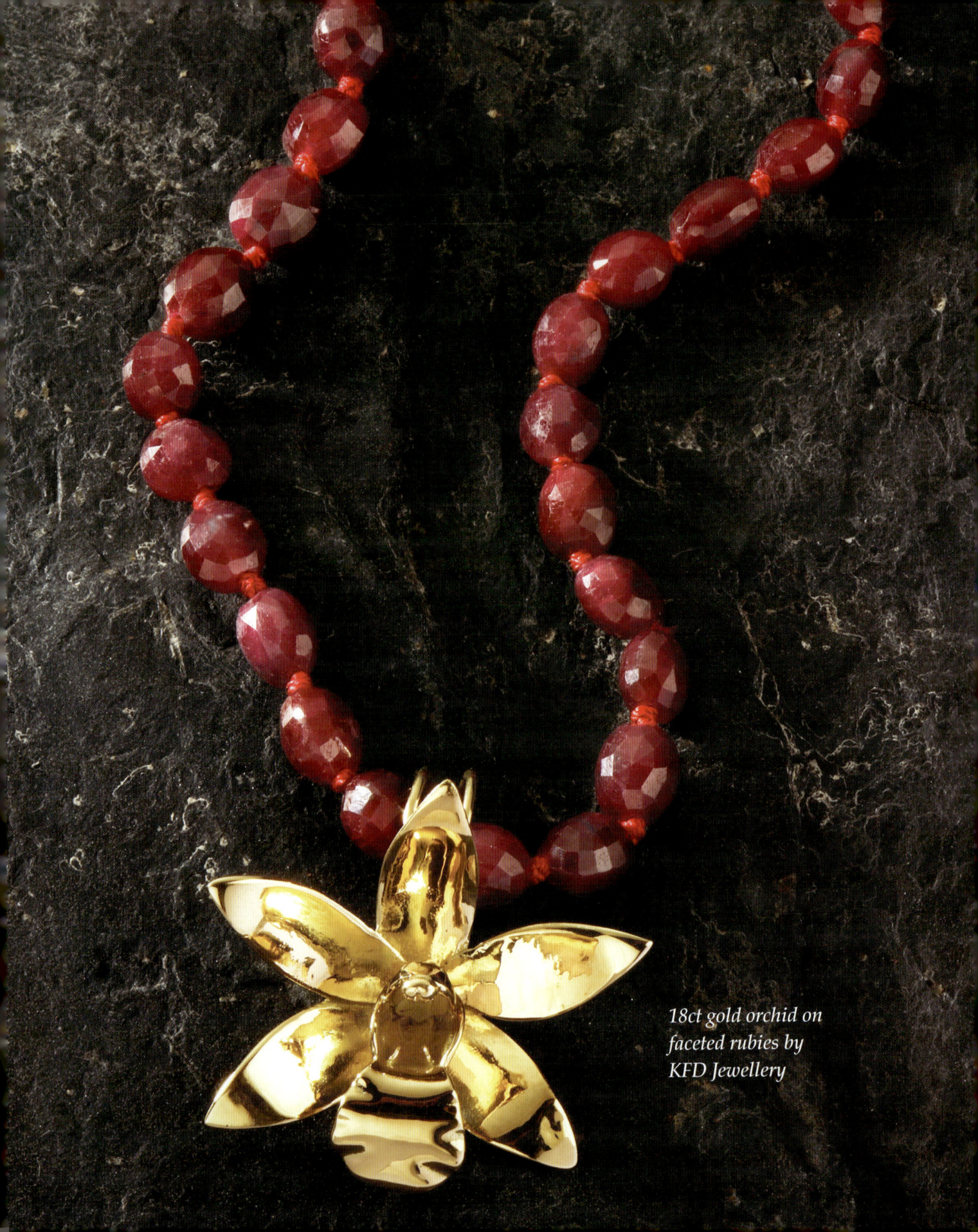

18ct gold orchid on faceted rubies by KFD Jewellery

About the Author

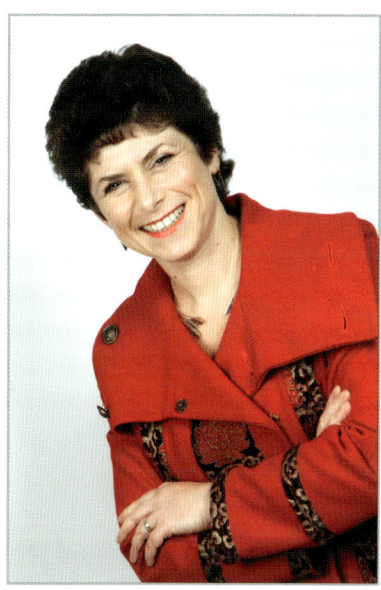

I graduated from Manchester Metropolitan University in 1987 with a BSc (Hons) in Biological Sciences. Following my marriage to Bruce in the summer of the same year, I started lecturing in biology on further and higher education courses in Manchester and Salford colleges. I continued teaching whilst raising our two children, Michael and Danielle. In 1999 I decided that I wanted to follow my passion for handmade jewellery, so I enrolled on a short evening course to study jewellery making and silversmithing. After re-locating to rural Cambridgeshire I started my second career path as a designer and maker of jewellery. Over the next few years I developed my skills on a series of short courses and master classes at the School of Jewellery at Birmingham University.

My interest in biology still prevails, as flowers and leaves inspire many of my jewellery collections. I work mainly in silver, but also use 9ct and 18ct gold. The jewellery exists in collections, with every collection having a statement necklace or torque as well as smaller pendants, earrings, bracelets and sometimes rings. The collections are designed to take the wearer through the day into the evening. I sell my work through a series of prestigious galleries and at shows around the UK.

I am a first-time author. My twelve years' experience designing, making, fitting and selling jewellery has given me a unique insight into the process of selecting the ideal piece of jewellery for the wearer. I have condensed this knowledge into an easy-to-read, easy reference format to guide you through the styles of jewellery to ensure that you always select the right collection for you, so that you look good, always.

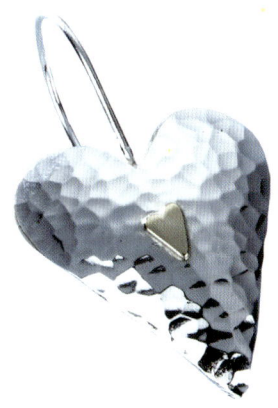

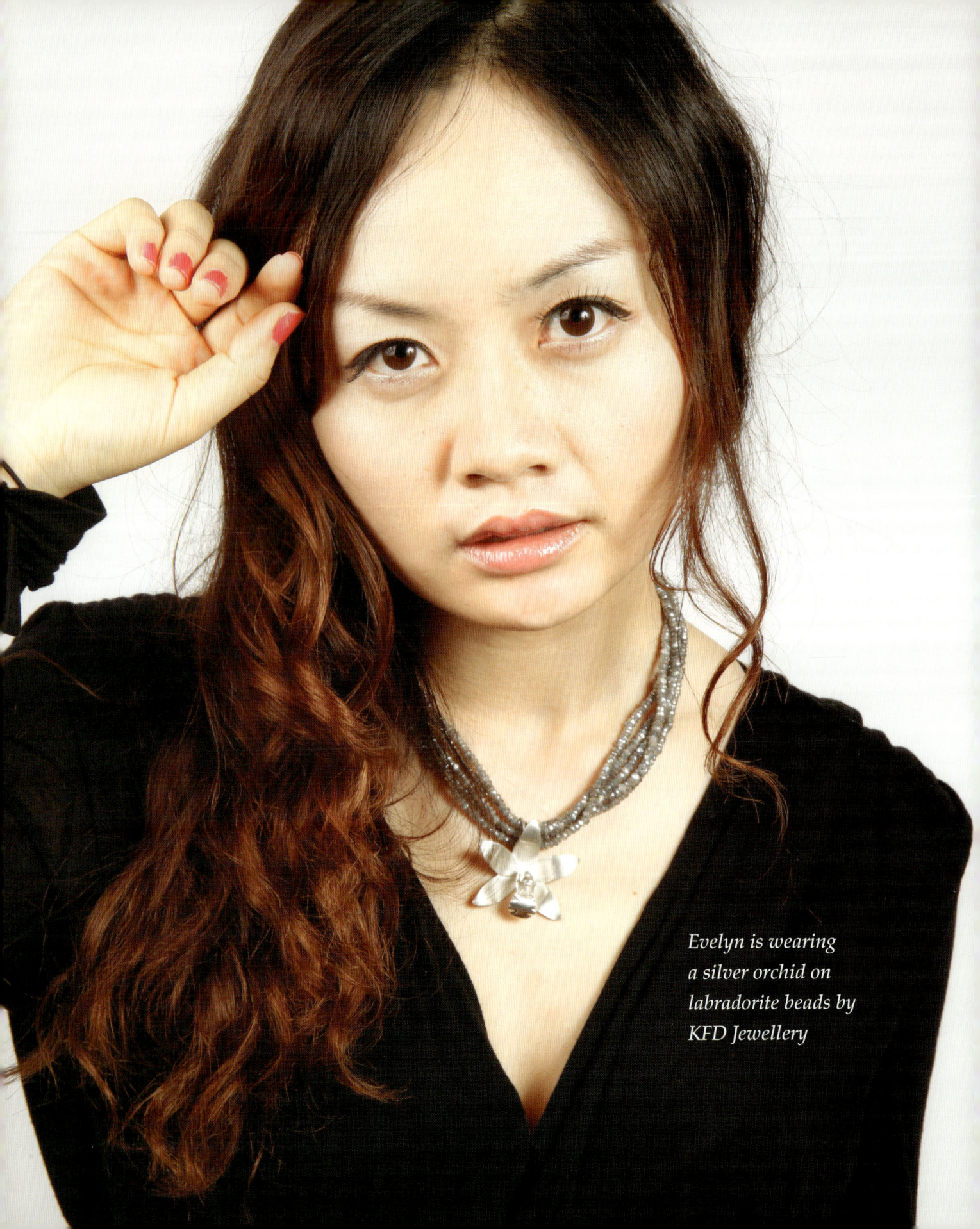

Evelyn is wearing a silver orchid on labradorite beads by KFD Jewellery

Introduction

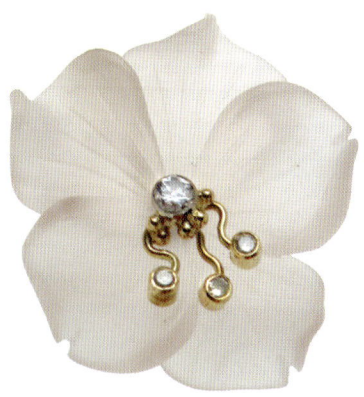

Wherever you are, whatever you're doing, you're judged on how you look. Image is important in both social and business environments. It is said that you have less than seven seconds to make a first impression, so it is essential that in these first few seconds you project a positive self image which is then maintained over subsequent meetings. The jewellery you wear is an important part of your persona – it can indicate your status, suggest your personality and hint at your occupation.

Throughout the ages, jewellery has been used to adorn the body. The oldest known jewellery, made from shell beads, is over 75,000 years old. Red ochre pigment was found on a necklace discovered in Blombos cave in South Africa. Is this evidence of early bead decoration or had the beads rubbed against the wearers' skin and picked up bits of early make-up?

Jewellery has served all sorts of different functions over time, from being simply practical – buckles, pins, clasps - through being a very convenient way of carrying your wealth around (and showing it off, of course), to magical or religious protection (amulets and magical symbols), and, finally, being a way of stating your membership of a particular group or organization.

Nowadays jewellery is used to signify love, as in an engagement ring or a wedding band, to celebrate an occasion such as a notable wedding anniversary, as a symbol of religion, to indicate wealth or as a fashion statement. Your choice of jewellery helps convey an impression of who you are.

Jewellery is made from a vast range of materials. Both inorganic materials such as metals, stone, glass, acrylics, plastics, and organic materials such as bone, wood, textiles, leather and feathers – the list is limited only by the imagination of the maker.

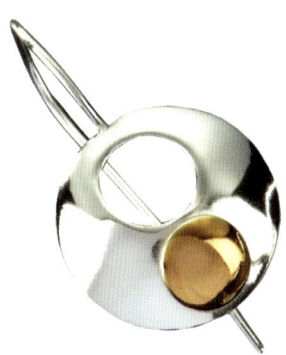

Jewellery is very personal, but there are a few guidelines that, if followed, can make you look good, always. This book aims to lead you through the process of choosing the jewellery to suit your physical characteristics, age, personality and the occasion for which you are wearing the jewellery. During your journey you will also be introduced to a selection of designer/maker jewellers from the UK, whose work has been used as examples throughout this book.

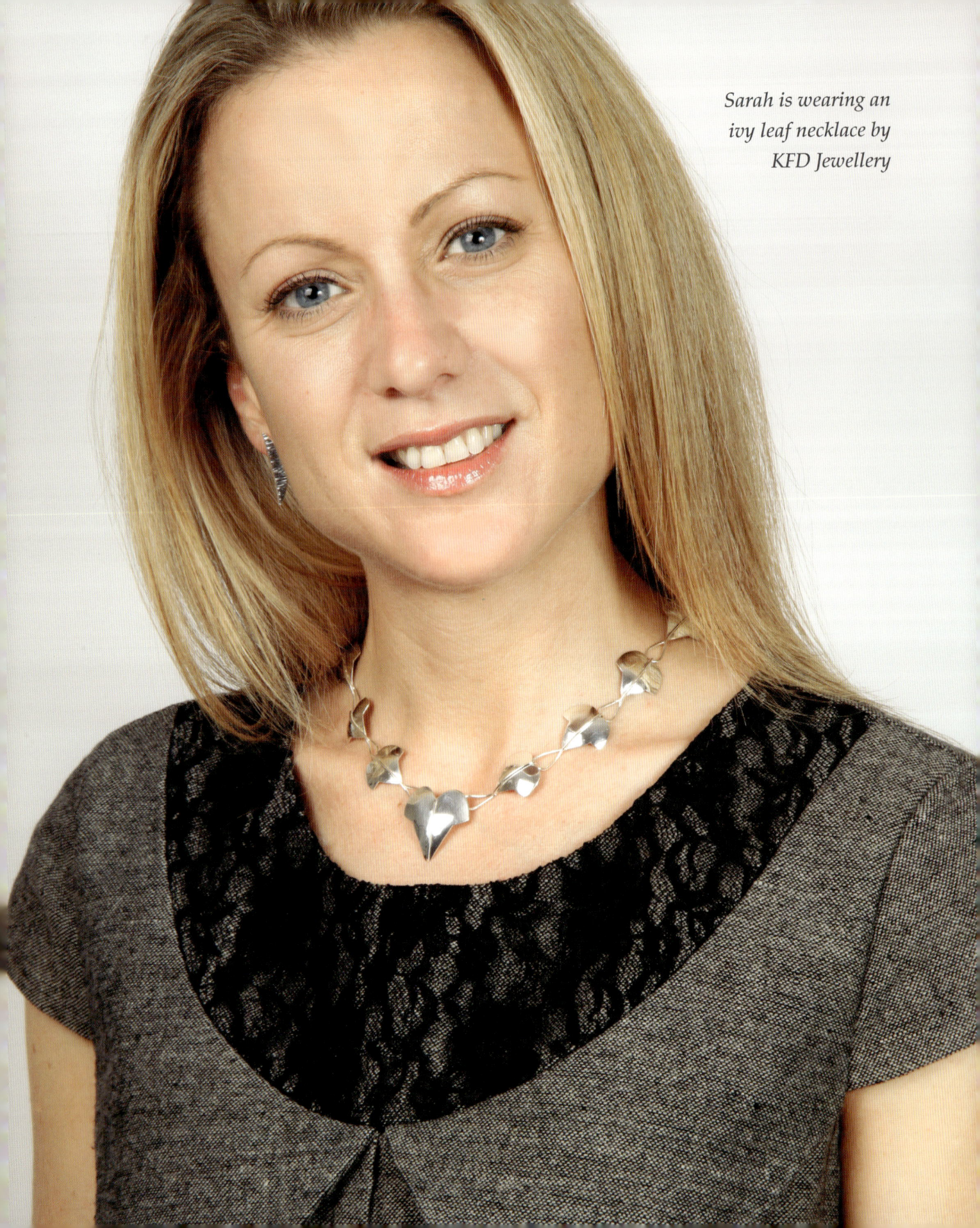

Sarah is wearing an ivy leaf necklace by KFD Jewellery

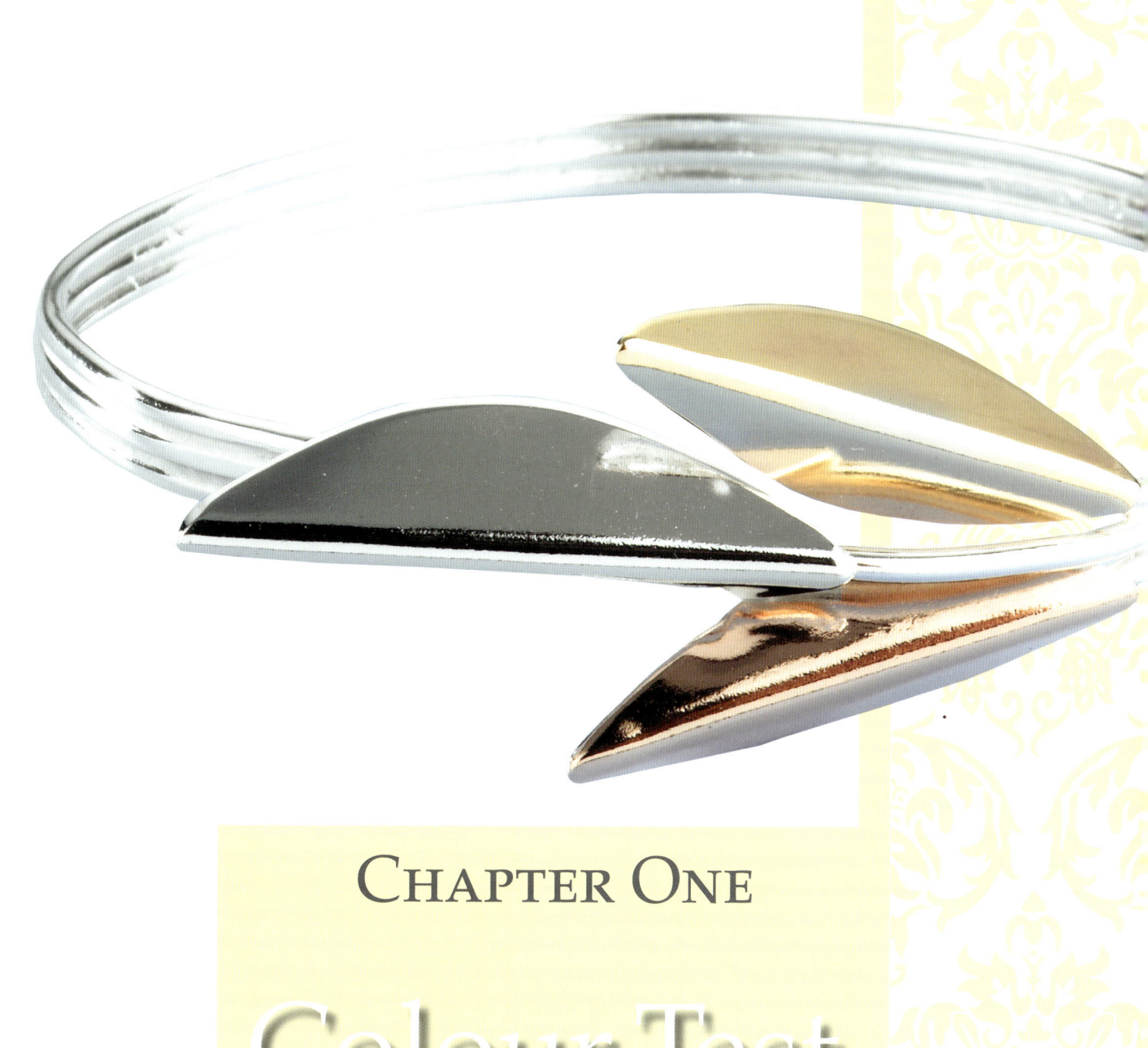

CHAPTER ONE

Colour Test

DOES THIS LOOK GOOD ON ME?

Colour Test

Skin tone, hair and eye colour are all important considerations when determining the colour palette that suits you. To look your best it is essential that you know your colours and wear those that harmonise with your natural colouring. There are a variety of companies and books on the market that guide you through this process. I have picked out a few that I think are particularly useful. They are listed on page 105. Wearing jewellery which is compatible with your colouring is vital to compliment your look.

When considering what jewellery to wear it is useful to first determine whether you are predominantly a silver or a gold person. This can be achieved by holding a series of metallic scarves close to the face and observing which looks best. Ideally this test should be carried out wearing no make-up. People who look better in silver tend to look sallow in gold tones. Those who suit gold tones look drained and pale next to silver.

To demonstrate this process a selection of scarves in silver, pewter, gold, copper and bronze were used with a group of models in order to determine their ideal metal colour.

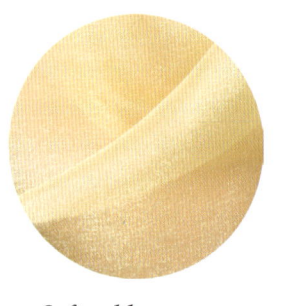
Soft gold

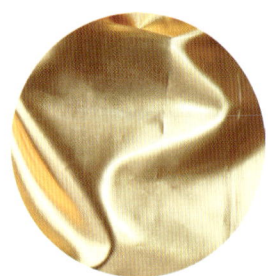
Clear gold

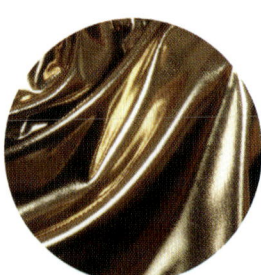
Dark gold

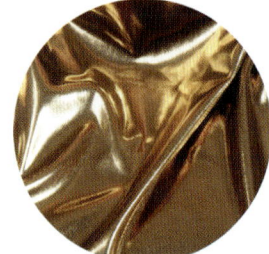
Bronze

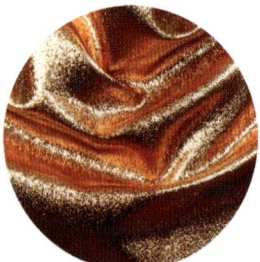
Copper

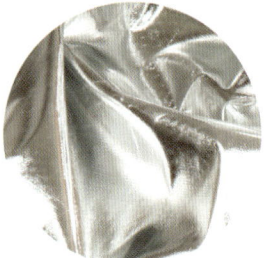
Silver

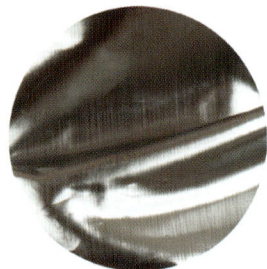
Pewter

CHAPTER ONE: COLOUR TEST

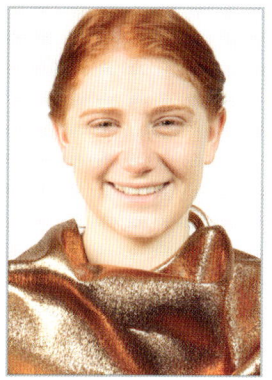
Copper

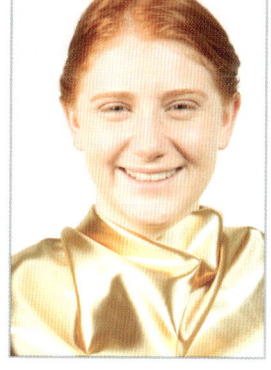
Clear gold

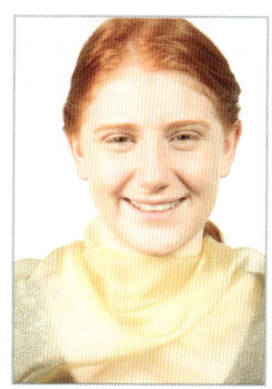
Soft gold

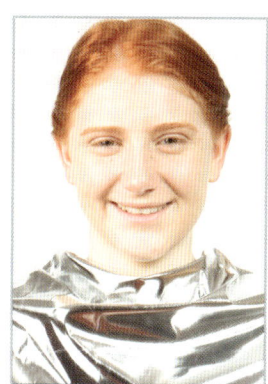
Silver

Danielle

The red hair of Danielle looks fabulous with the copper coloured scarf. Danielle also looks good in gold, but look how she becomes drained of colour when wrapped in the silver scarf. Danielle suits all gold, copper and bronze metals.

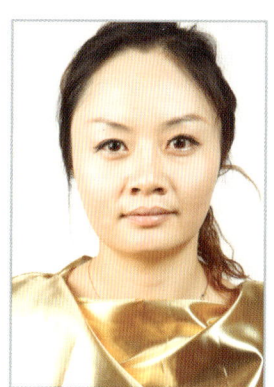
Clear gold

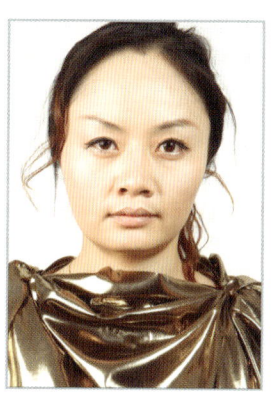
Dark gold

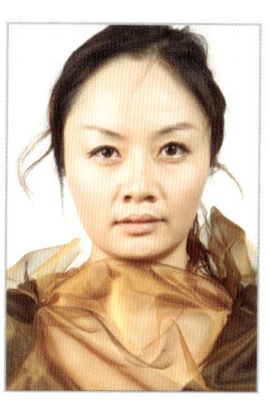
Soft gold

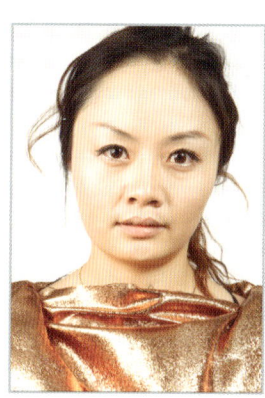
Copper

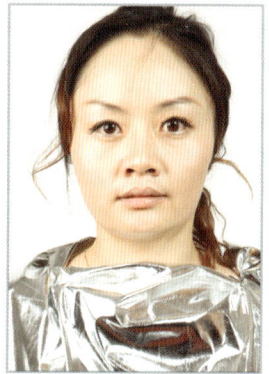
Silver

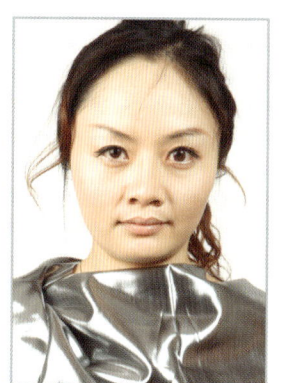
Pewter

Evelyn

Evelyn's black hair, warm brown eyes and yellowish skin tone look good with a clear gold colour. She can carry other shades of gold, but the copper scarf is not flattering with Evelyn's skin tone. The silver and pewter scarves drain her skin.

11

Does This Look Good On Me?

Helena

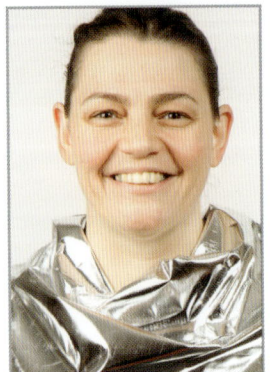
Silver

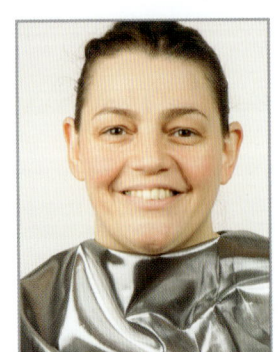
Pewter

Sarah

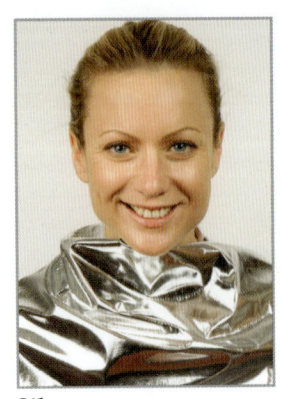
Silver

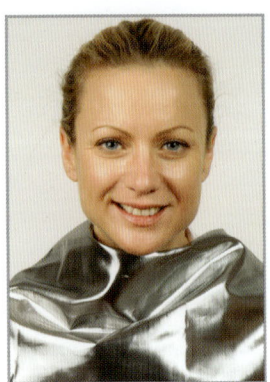
Pewter

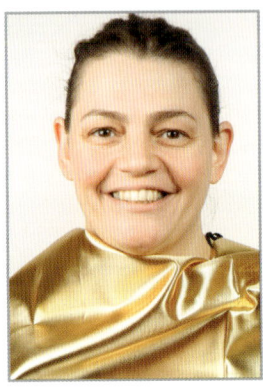
Clear gold

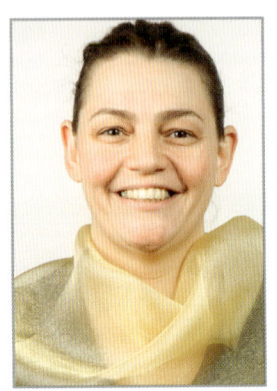
Soft gold

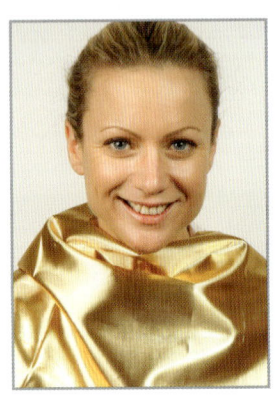
Clear gold

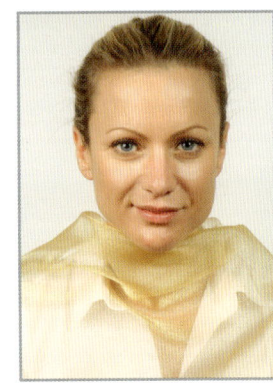
Soft gold

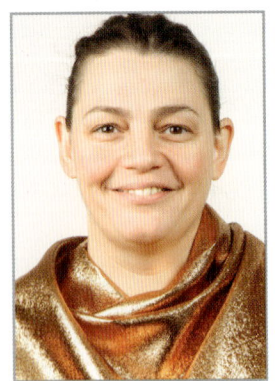
Copper

Both Sarah and Helena's skin show shadows and look sallow with the gold, bronze and copper scarves, but look brighter with the silver scarf. The pewter scarf is not ideal for Helena or Sarah; they are both clear silver people.

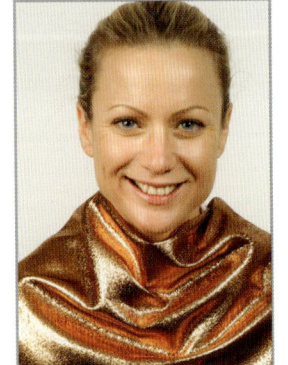
Copper

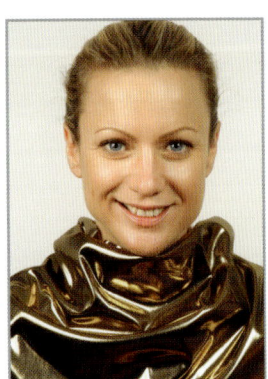
Dark gold

CHAPTER ONE: COLOUR TEST

Jade

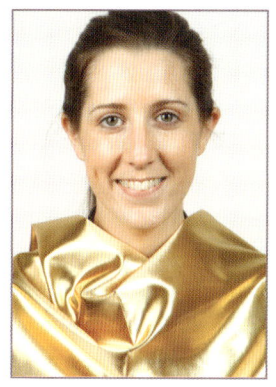
Clear gold

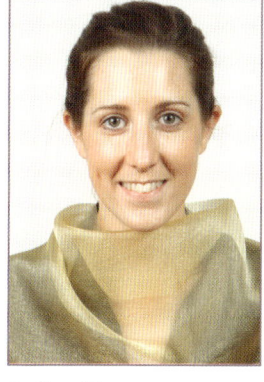
Soft gold

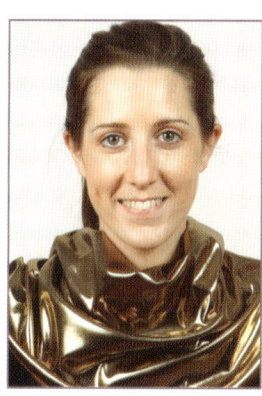
Dark gold

Jade's golden brown hair, hazel eyes and freckled skin came alive with the bronze and gold scarves. The copper scarf was not as good as the gold, but considerably better than the silver scarves which drained her face and made her look pale.

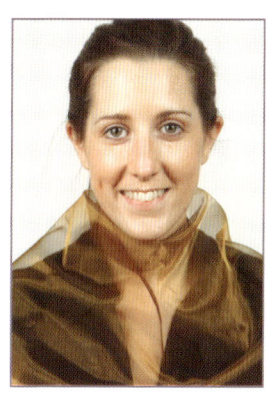
Bronze

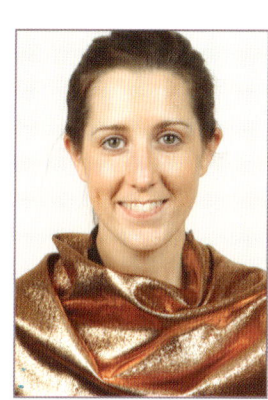
Copper

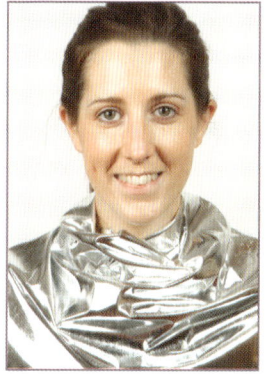
Silver

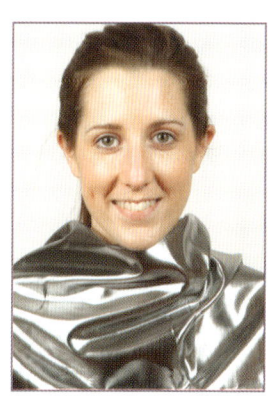
Pewter

Does This Look Good On Me?

Beverley

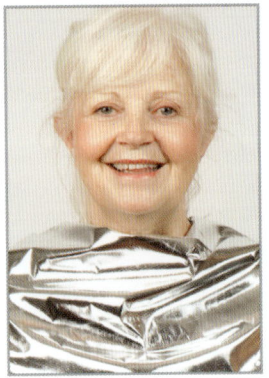
Silver

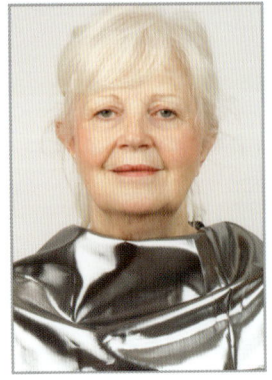
Pewter

Beverley's white hair, bright blue eyes and pale skin might have suggested that she suits silver rather than gold, however the scarf test produced some surprising results. Whilst the bronze and dark gold scarves were not flattering to Beverley's skin tone, she did look good in the clear gold as well as in the silver scarves. This will be discussed further in the following chapters.

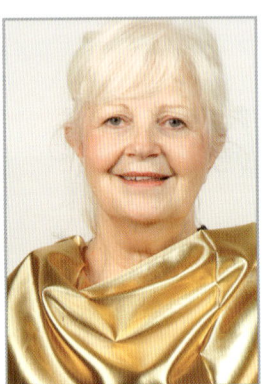
Clear gold

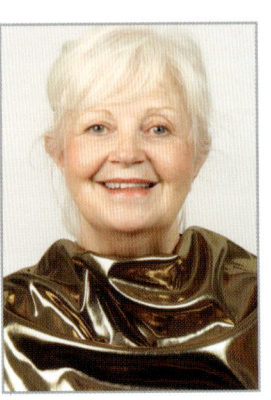
Dark gold

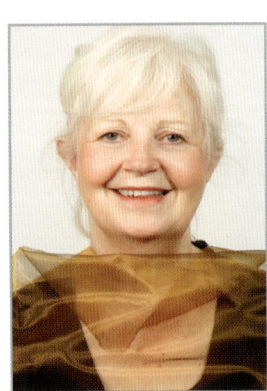
Bronze

It can therefore be seen that although you will have a dominance of either silver or gold in your colouring, you will not necessarily suit all shades of gold or silver. There are a variety of silver and gold coloured metals on the jewellery market and so it should be relatively easy to find the ideal metal for both your colouring and your budget

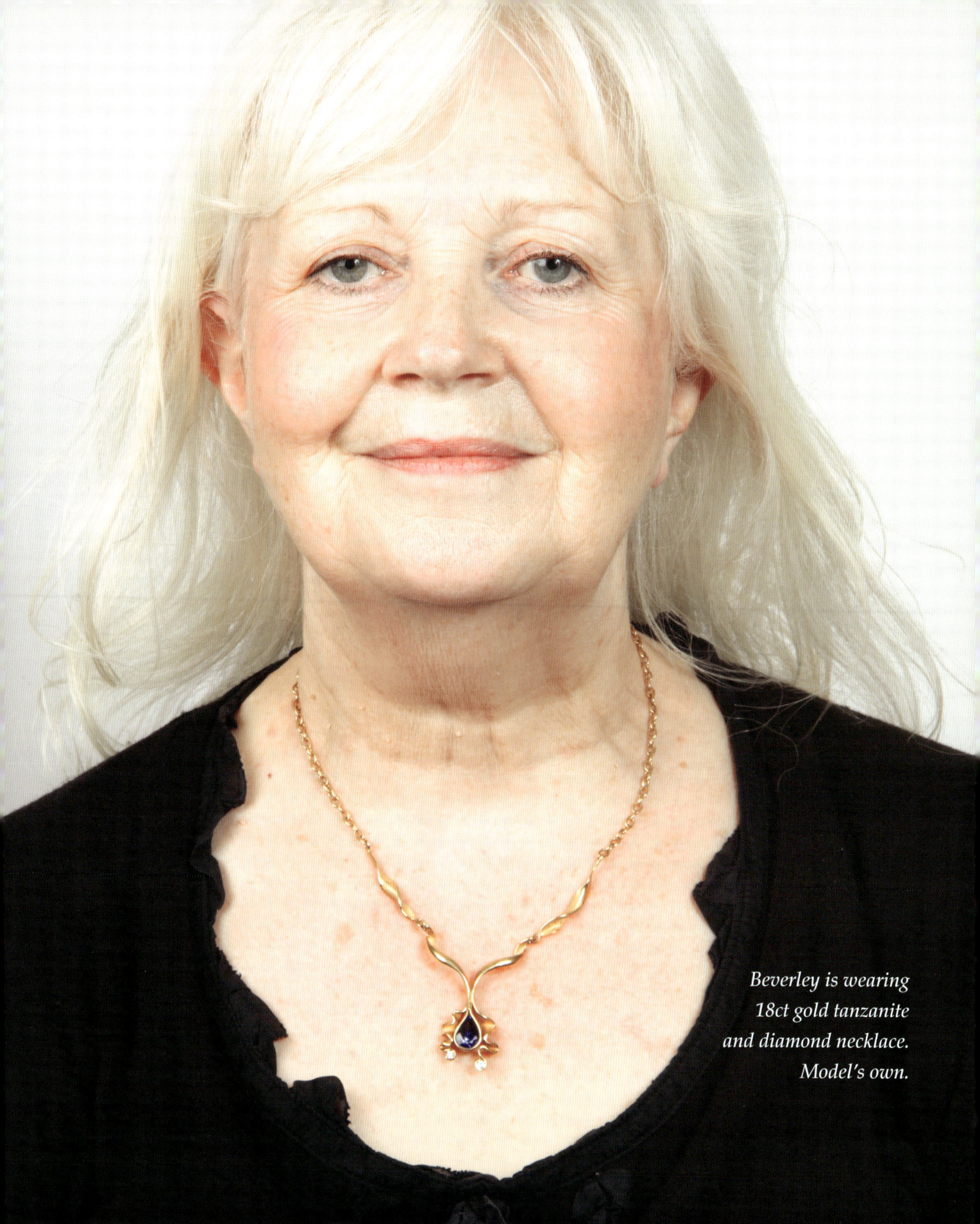

Beverley is wearing 18ct gold tanzanite and diamond necklace. Model's own.

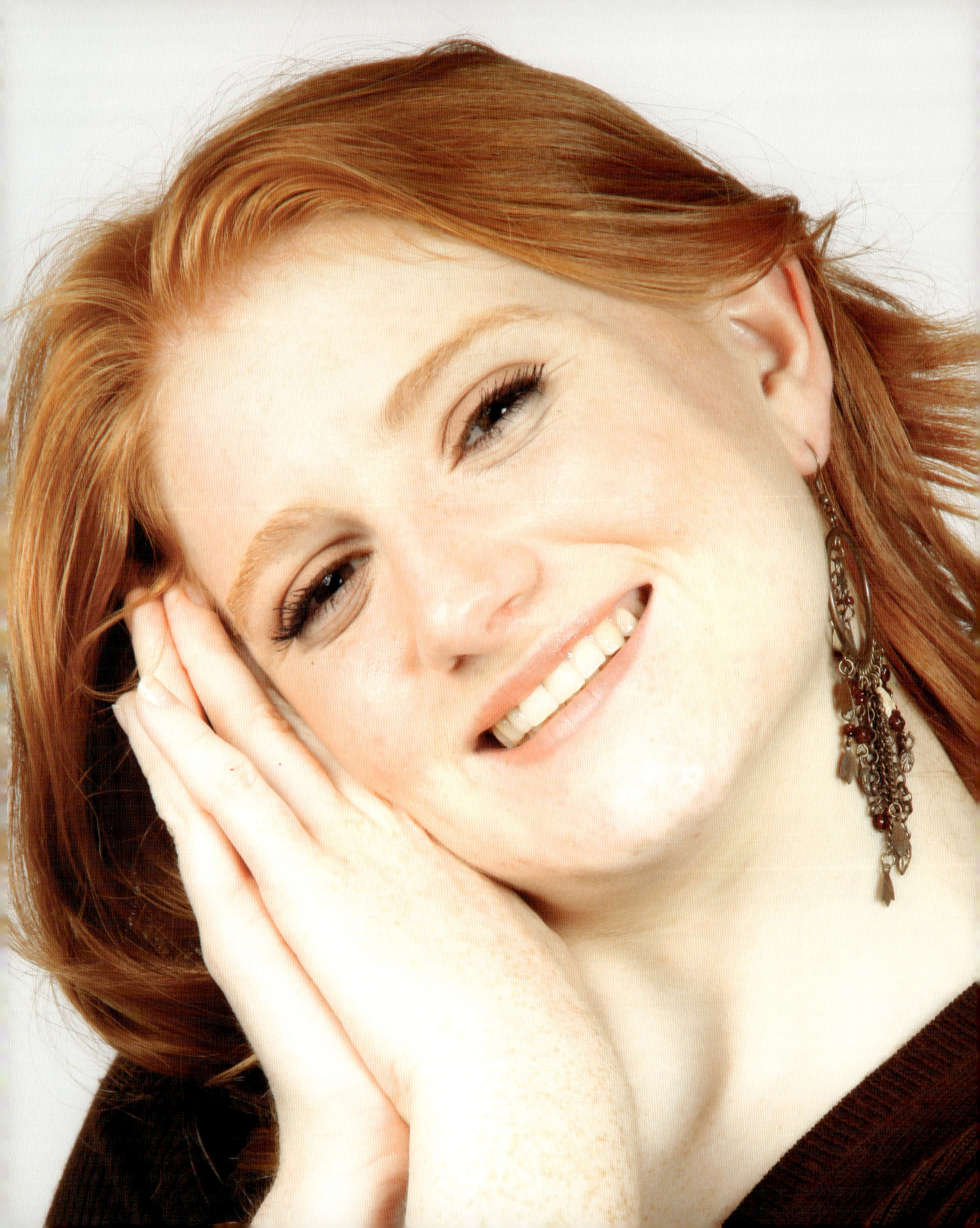

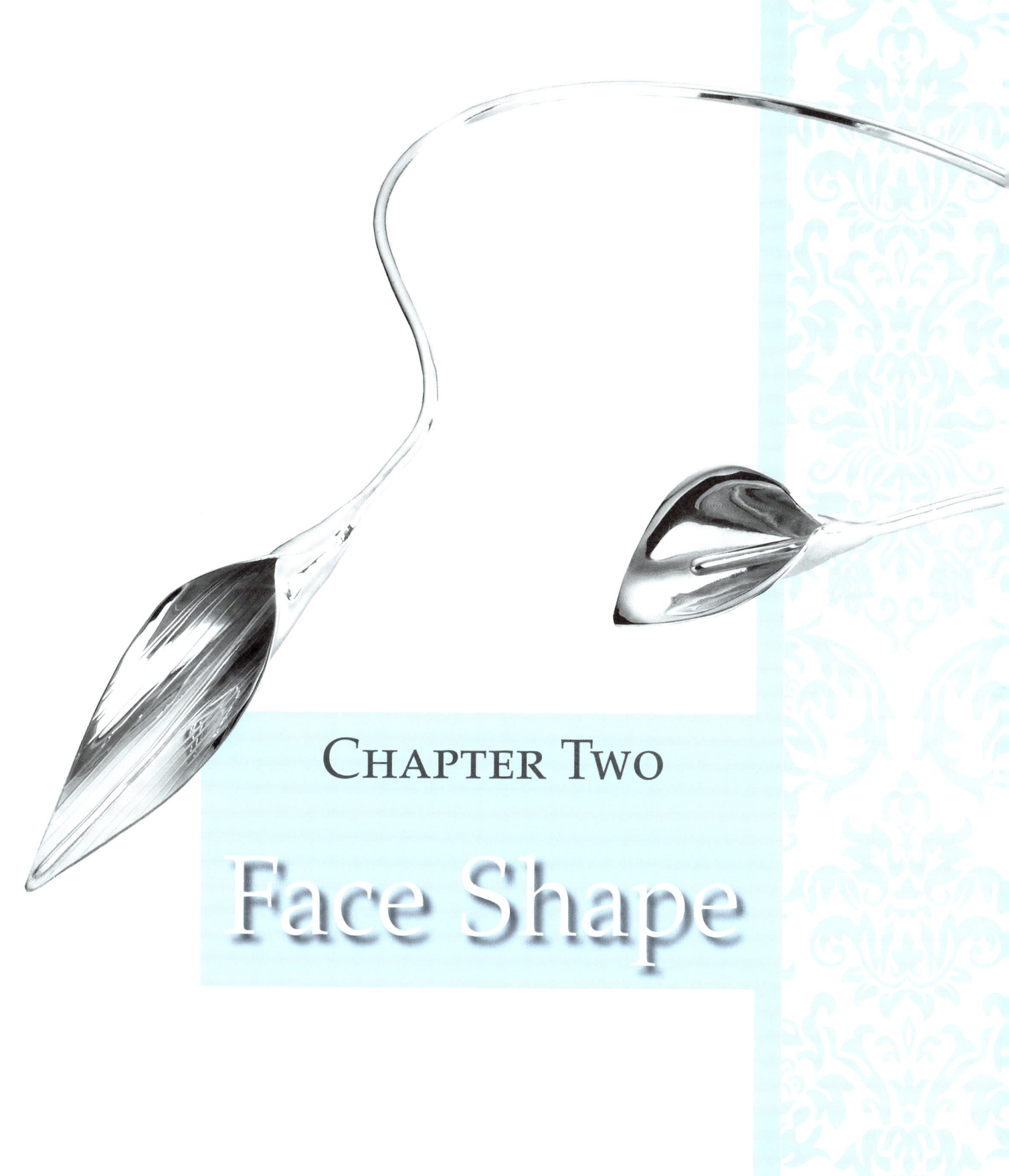

Chapter Two

Face Shape

Does This Look Good On Me?

Face Shape

Face shape and characteristics vary considerably from person to person. Facial features give you an identity and make you unique. The oval face shape, with its well balanced features, is the shape which most people in the West consider to be the ideal. It is possible to emphasise and draw attention to the good points of a face with the correct choice of earrings.

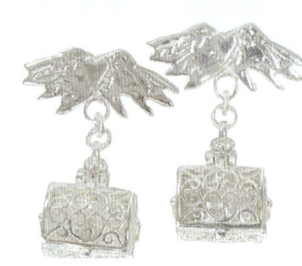

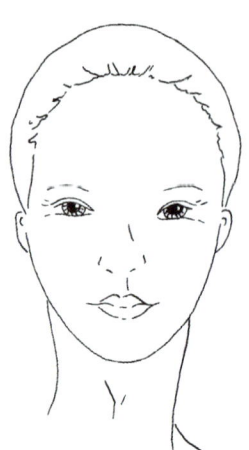

Oval

This is a balanced, in proportion, versatile face, with no extreme characteristics. Your face is slightly longer in length than width and your chin is softly rounded.

Jewellery Notes
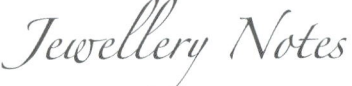

This is the ideal face shape which suits any type of earrings, although it would be good to avoid very long earrings if your neck is short.

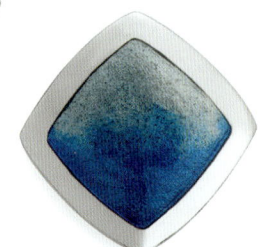

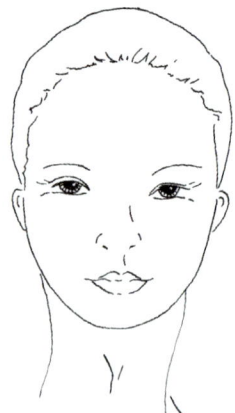

Round

The length and width of your face are almost equal and your jaw rounded. Your cheekbones are the widest part of your face

Jewellery Notes
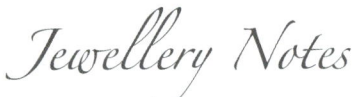

Earrings can be used to lengthen the face. Oval or long thin shapes are good. Dangly earrings are good if your neck is long. Avoid round earrings as these will add width to your face.

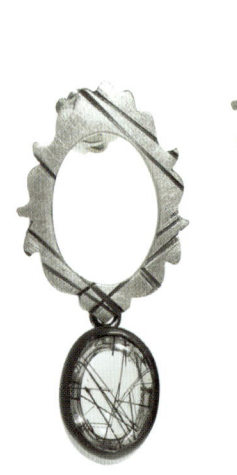
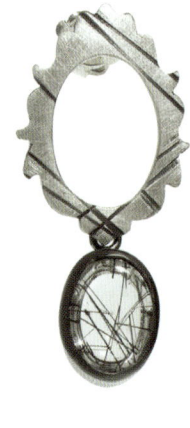

CHAPTER TWO: FACE SHAPE

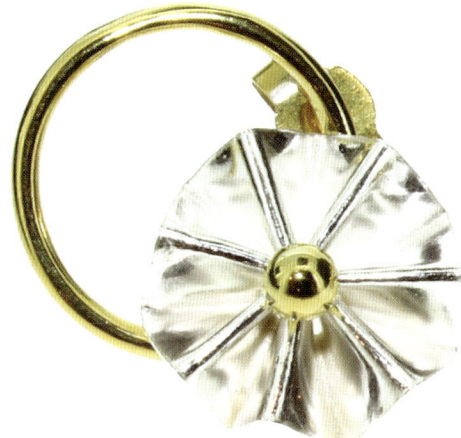

Rectangle

Your face is long and thin and you have a fairly square jawline. Your forehead, cheekbones and jawline are equal widths.

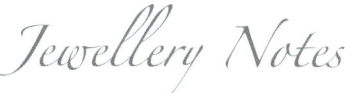

Earrings can be used to shorten the face. Round earrings are good, but avoid angular earrings which will exaggerate your jawline. Long dangly earring are also best avoided as these lengthen your face.

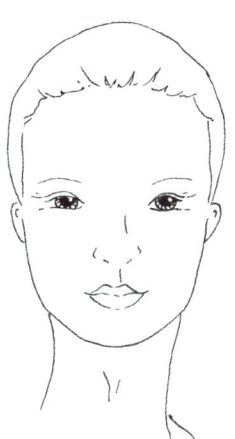

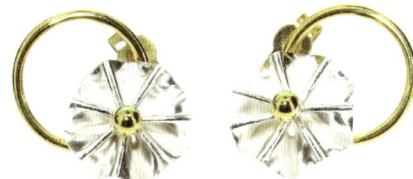

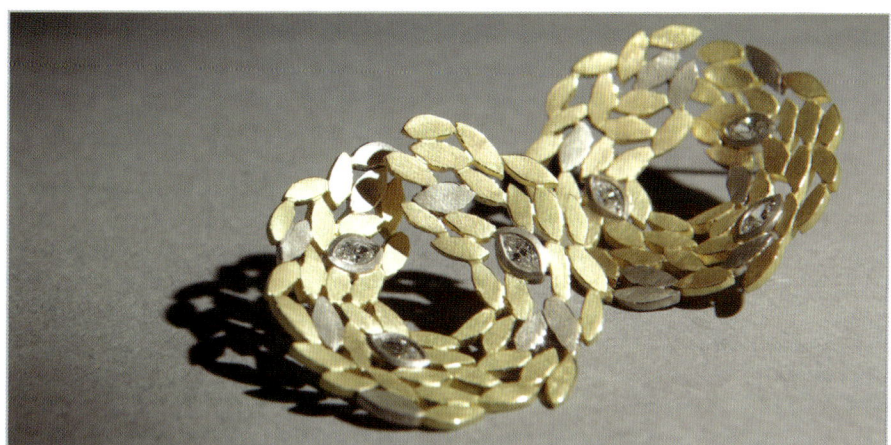

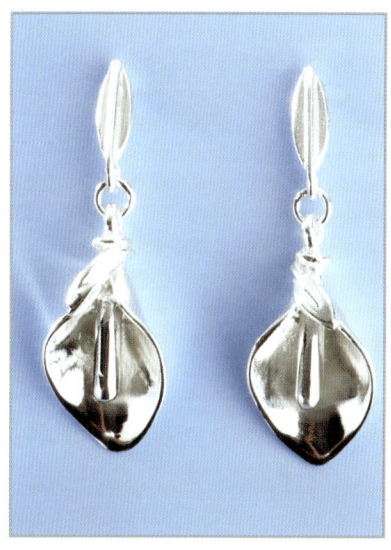

Oblong

Your face is long and thin and your jawline is softly rounded. Your forehead, cheekbones and jawline are equal widths.

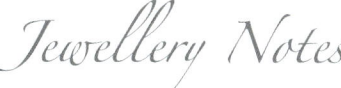

Earrings can be used to shorten the face. Round and curvaceous earrings are good. Avoid long thin dangly earrings. Short drop earrings (to mouth level only) could add width and give the illusion of reducing the length of the face.

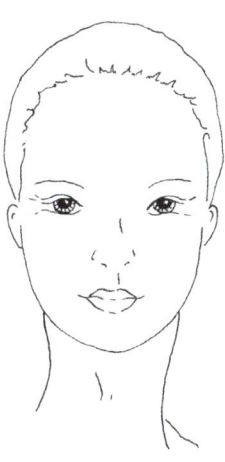

19

Does This Look Good On Me?

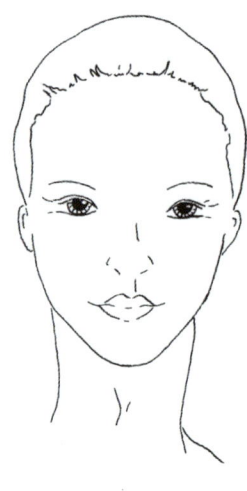

Inverted triangle

Your face is slightly longer in length than width. The widest part of your face is the forehead, although the cheekbones may be the same width. Your jaw is the narrowest part of your face.

Jewellery Notes

Your desirable jawline can be emphasised with larger earrings. Show off your good features by wearing dangly earrings if you have a long neck.

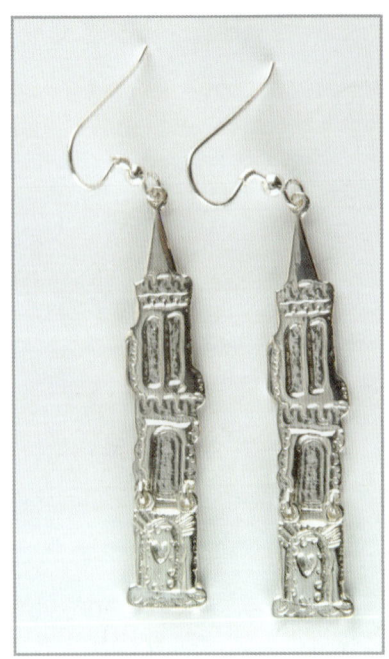

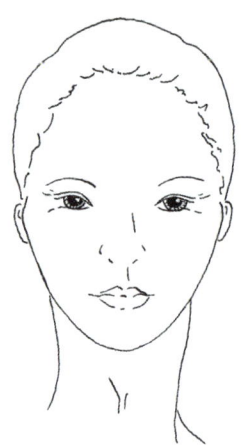

Diamond

The face is slightly longer in length than width and the chin is long and pointed. The cheekbones are the widest part of the face.

Jewellery Notes

Larger earrings are good to draw attention to your jawline. Long, dangly earrings are fabulous for you so long as you have a long neck.

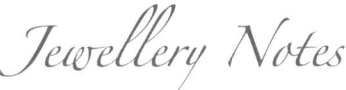
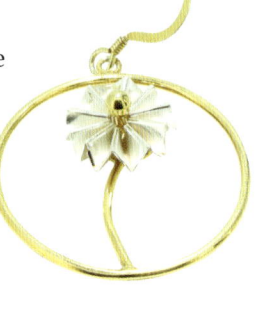
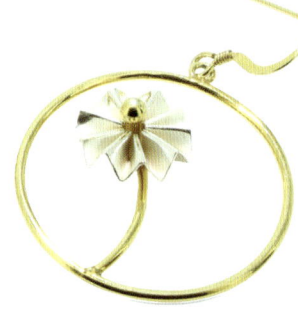
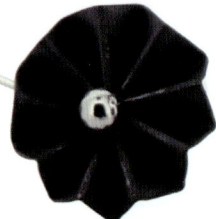
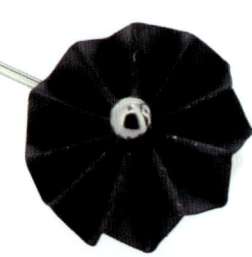
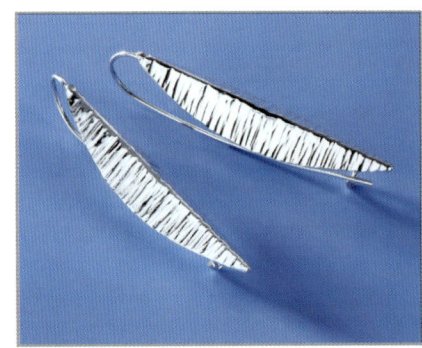

20

CHAPTER TWO: FACE SHAPE

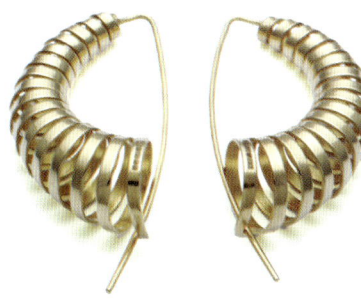

Heart shaped

Your face has similar features to the inverted triangle only your hairline has the characteristic 'widow's peak'.

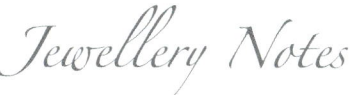

Wear larger earrings to highlight your good jawline. If you have a long neck you can also emphasise this by wearing dangly earrings.

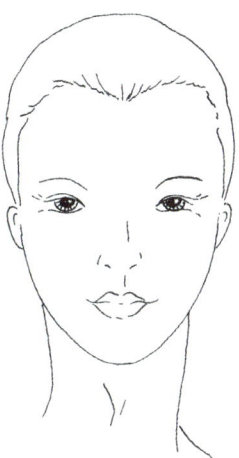

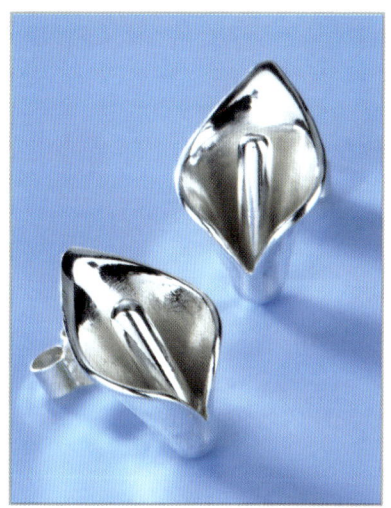

Square

The length and width of your face are almost equal.

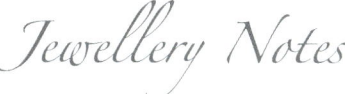

Rounded shaped earrings are good, but avoid angular earrings which will emphasise the angles on your face. Avoid earrings which end at your jawline.

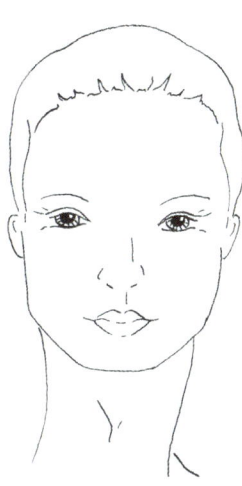

Triangle

Your face is slightly longer in length than width. Your forehead is the narrowest part of the face and your jawline the widest.

Jewellery Notes

Rounded shaped earrings are good, but avoid angular earrings which will emphasise the angles on your face. Avoid earrings which end at your jawline.

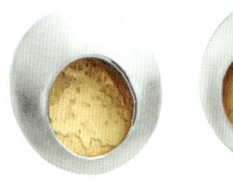
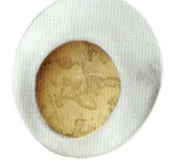
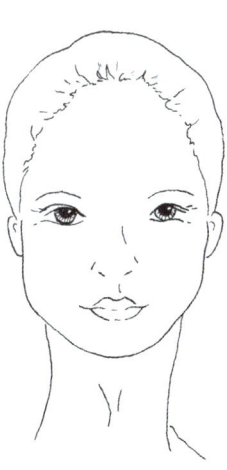

21

DOES THIS LOOK GOOD ON ME?

Neck length

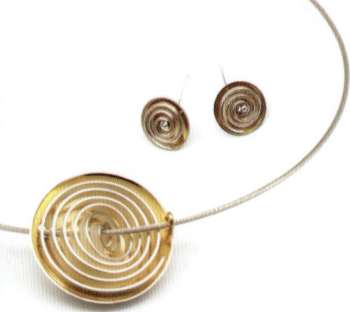

Once you have identified your face shape, take a look at your neck length and width. The general rule of thumb is that if you have a short neck, or a particularly wide neck, avoid dangly earrings. If you really love long earrings, but do not have a long neck, try shorter length drop earrings that hang just below the ear lobe.

If you are lucky enough to have a long, slender neck then you are in the fortunate position to be able to wear necklaces of any length. Ideally draw attention to this desirable feature by wearing a choker, a collar, torque or other short necklace. If your neck is short or wide then it is best that you avoid choker or shorter length necklaces and opt instead for a necklace midway between your neck and your breast. Alternatively choose a brooch and position it appropriately – your focal point should be midway between your breast and neck.

Build of body

Another consideration when deciding on your jewellery choice is your body frame size. If you are very petite, then you will generally be better with small, delicate jewellery which will not overpower your small frame. If you have a larger frame then you will need to consider chunkier, more substantial jewellery which will not be lost on you.

If your bust size is very small or very large then you need to choose your necklace style carefully. The very small chested person can disguise this fact by choosing a very long necklace such as a long string of pearls or beads, which draws the eye down the length of the torso, not focusing on any one area in particular. The large chested lady does not have this option as strings of beads or a long pendant will not hang correctly over her bust, thereby unintentionally drawing attention to this area.

Age

As we age our skin undergoes a variety of changes, one of which is the loss of elasticity and tone. This results in the loose skin contributing to 'turkey neck', sagging skin around the jawline and 'droopy' ear lobes. Consequently, as you age, it is advisable not to emphasise these areas. Dangly earrings, especially those with hook fittings, will exaggerate droopy ear lobes and any sagging skin around the jawline. Short, thin chains should be avoided, with longer pendants being preferrable. Statement collar type necklaces might be a good option instead of wearing higher necklines and scarves. Brooches are also a good alternative to necklaces.

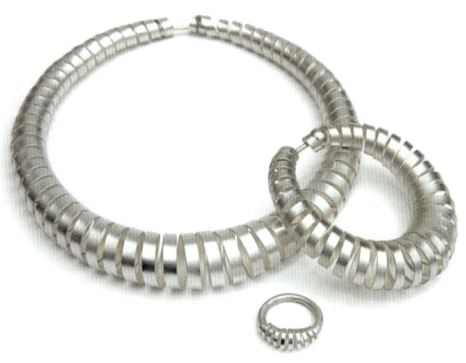

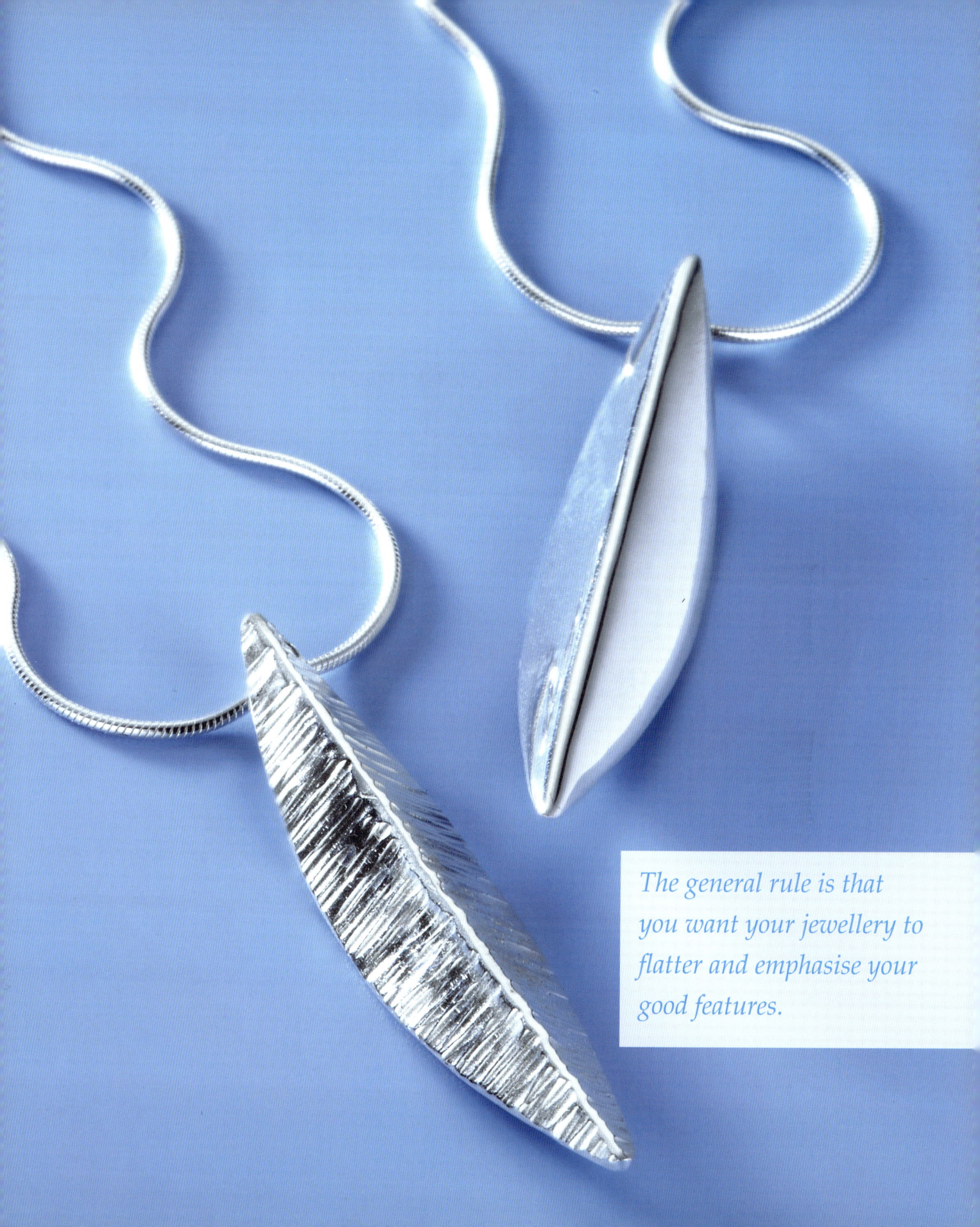

The general rule is that you want your jewellery to flatter and emphasise your good features.

Does This Look Good On Me?

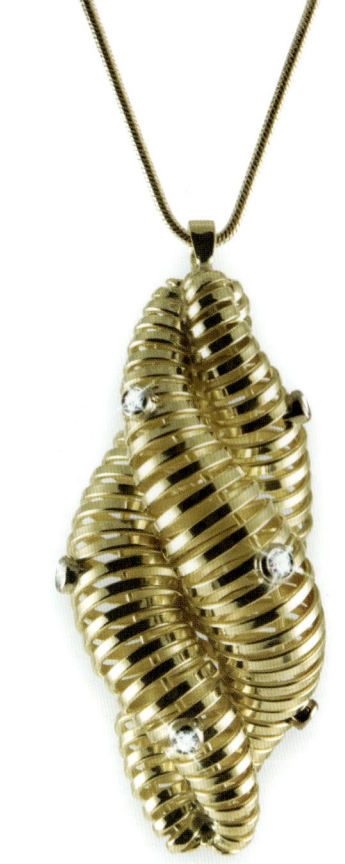

Danielle

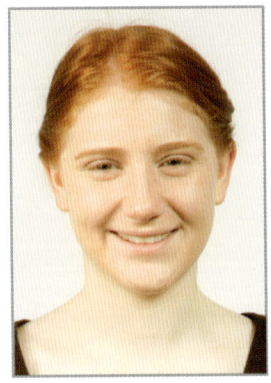

Danielle has a roundish oval face, her forehead is too narrow to be a true oval. Most styles of earring and necklace will suit her.

Danielle has a slender, longish neck so can therefore wear any style of necklace.

Evelyn

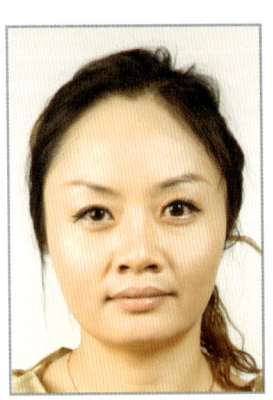

Evelyn's face shape is fairly diamond like, but she has a round jawline. Smaller earrings and thin, dangly earrings would be advisable. Dangly earrings should be shorter and not finish on her jawline.

Evelyn has a slim but relatively short neck, therefore would be best to avoid choker style necklaces.

Beverley

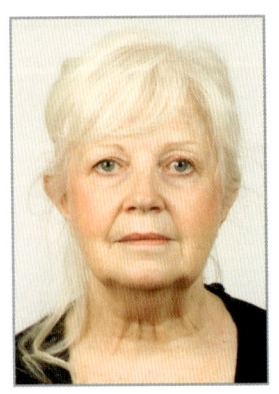

Beverley has a fairly well proportioned oval bone structure. Beverley wears both stud and drop earrings. The ideal earring length for Beverley would be mouth level.

As a slightly older lady, necklaces which focus the eye to mid chest height and away from the neck would be most suitable for Beverley.

CHAPTER TWO: FACE SHAPE

Helena

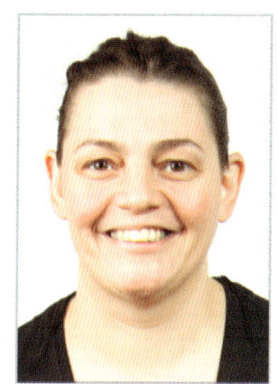

Helena has a round face, so round earrings would not be ideal. Angular earrings would be good as would be shorter, slimline drop earrings.

Necklaces which focus attention on the mid part of the chest are ideal for Helena.

Sarah

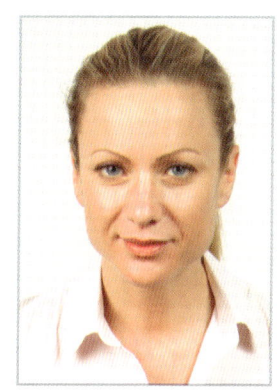

Sarah has an inverted triangle face shape, but with a fairly square jawline, which is the same width as her forehead. Smaller stud earrings with rounded shapes are ideal. Sarah can also wear dangly earrings, but they must end below or well above her jawline to deflect attention from this area.

Sarah has a long, slender neck, and so she can wear any style of necklace.

Jade

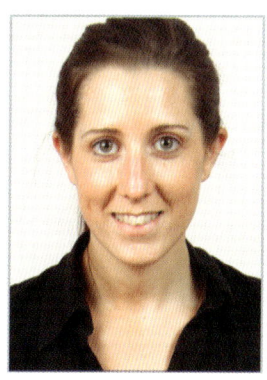

Jade has an oblong face and therefore suits rounded stud earrings. Long thin dangly earrings would emphasize the length of Jade's face.

Jade has a long slender neck, so can wear most styles of necklace.

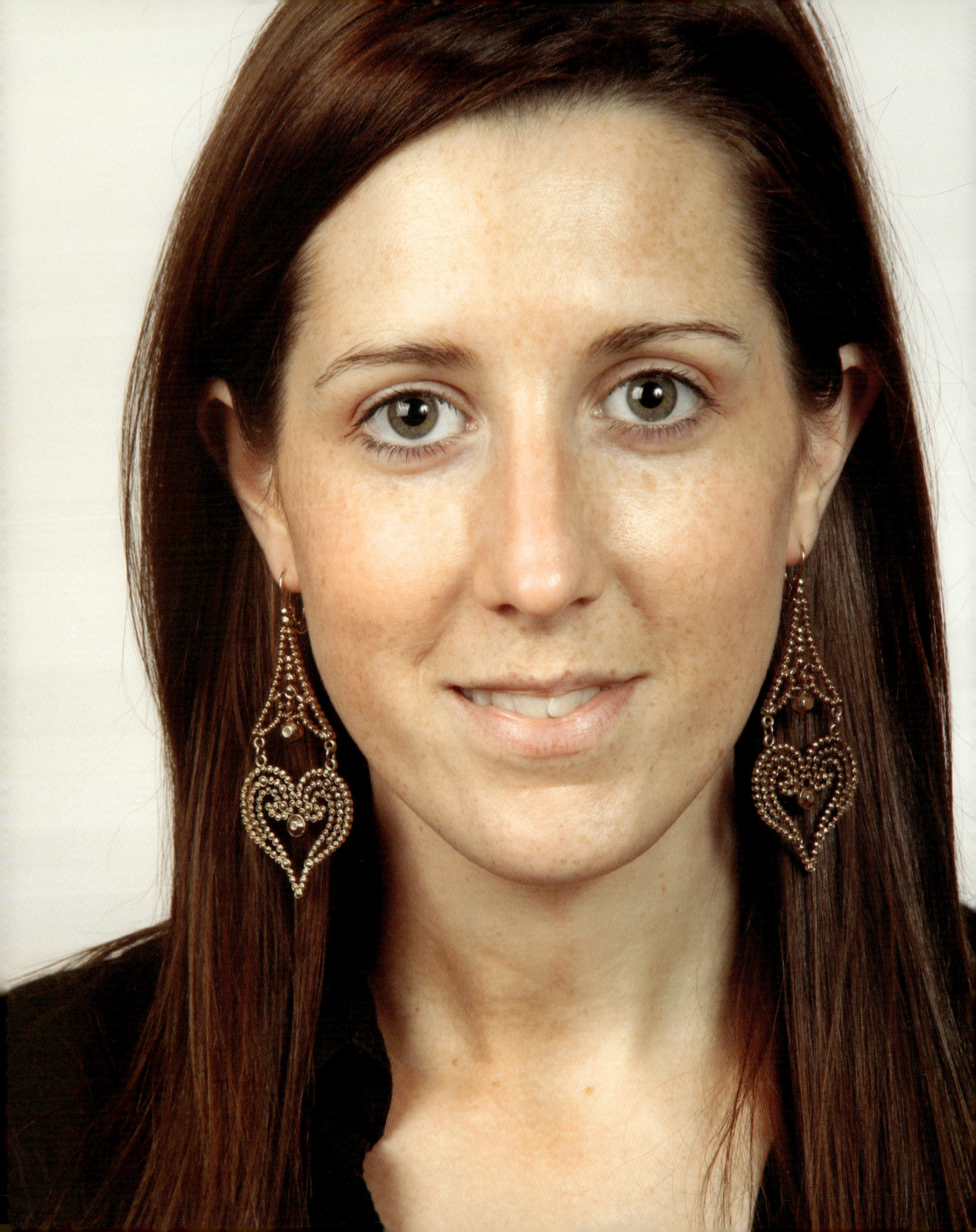

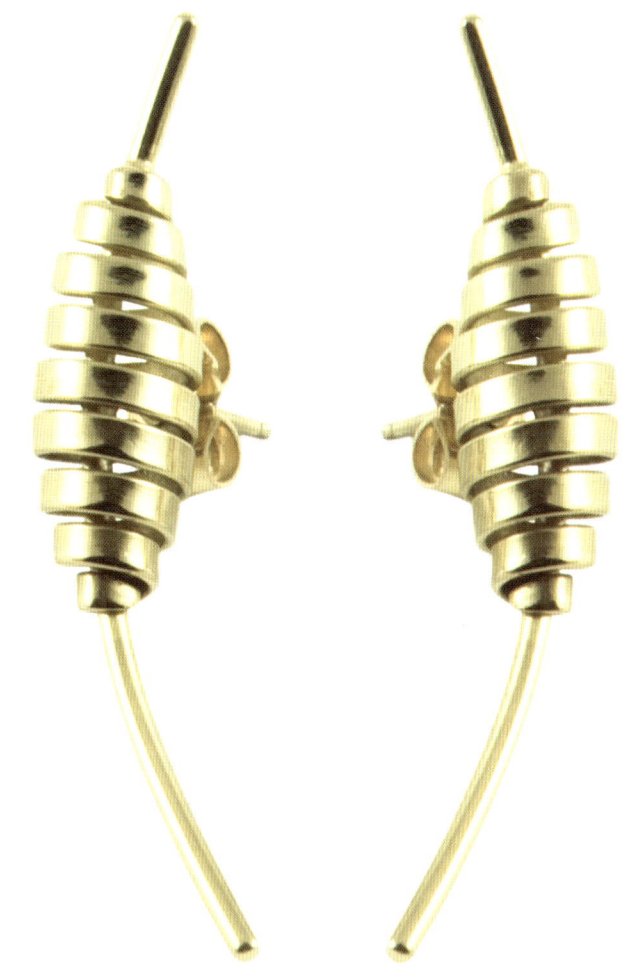

Chapter Three

Earrings & Face Shape

DOES THIS LOOK GOOD ON ME?

Earrings & Face Shape

Jade has an oblong face which means that round stud earrings are best for her. Long dangly earrings will tend to make her face appear longer and thinner.

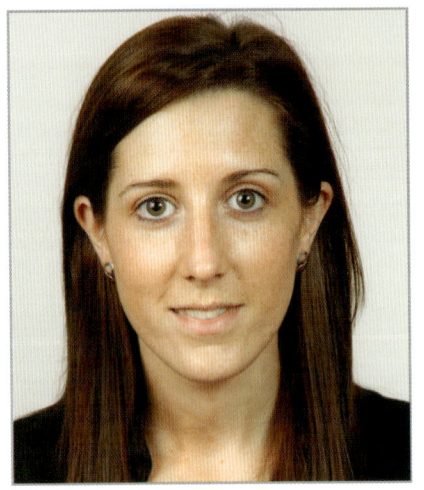

These round stud earrings flatter her face shape, however Jade suits gold better than silver, therefore would look better in gold coloured round stud earrings.

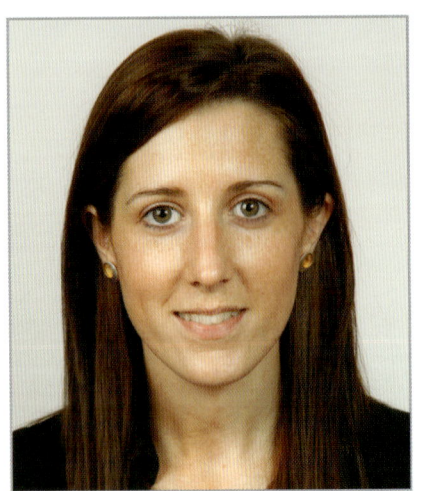

These earrings are a similar size to the previous earrings, but have a larger area of 18 ct gold plate, and so they suit Jade's colouring much better.

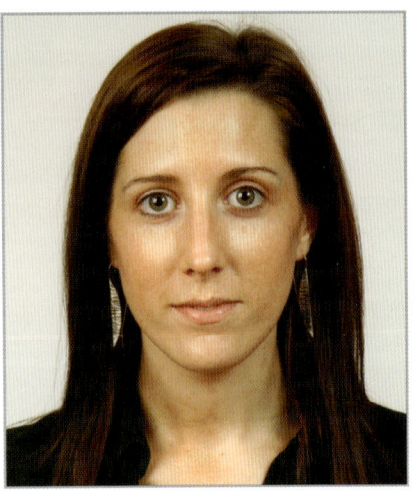

These long thin earrings are not suitable for Jade as they lengthen her face and, as they are silver as opposed to gold, they make her look pale.

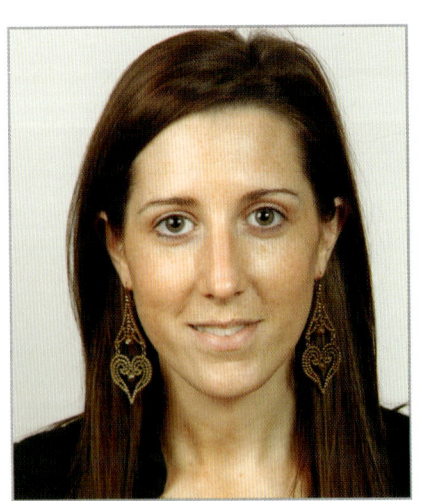

Although Jades's face shape is not ideally suited to long earrings, these do work as they draw the eye to the soft curve of her jawline while adding some width to her face.

CHAPTER THREE: EARRINGS & FACE SHAPE

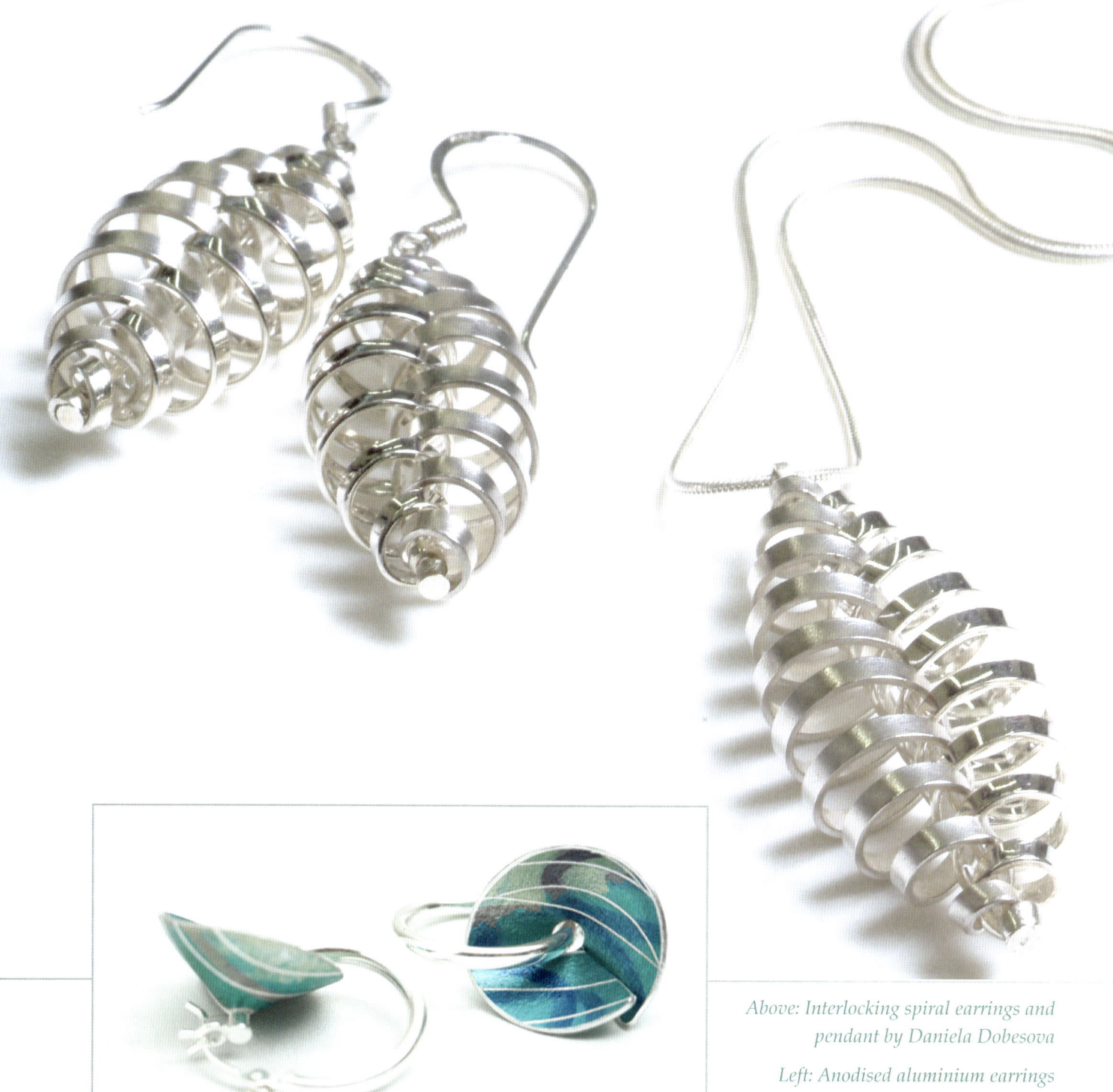

Above: Interlocking spiral earrings and pendant by Daniela Dobesova

Left: Anodised aluminium earrings by Carole Allen

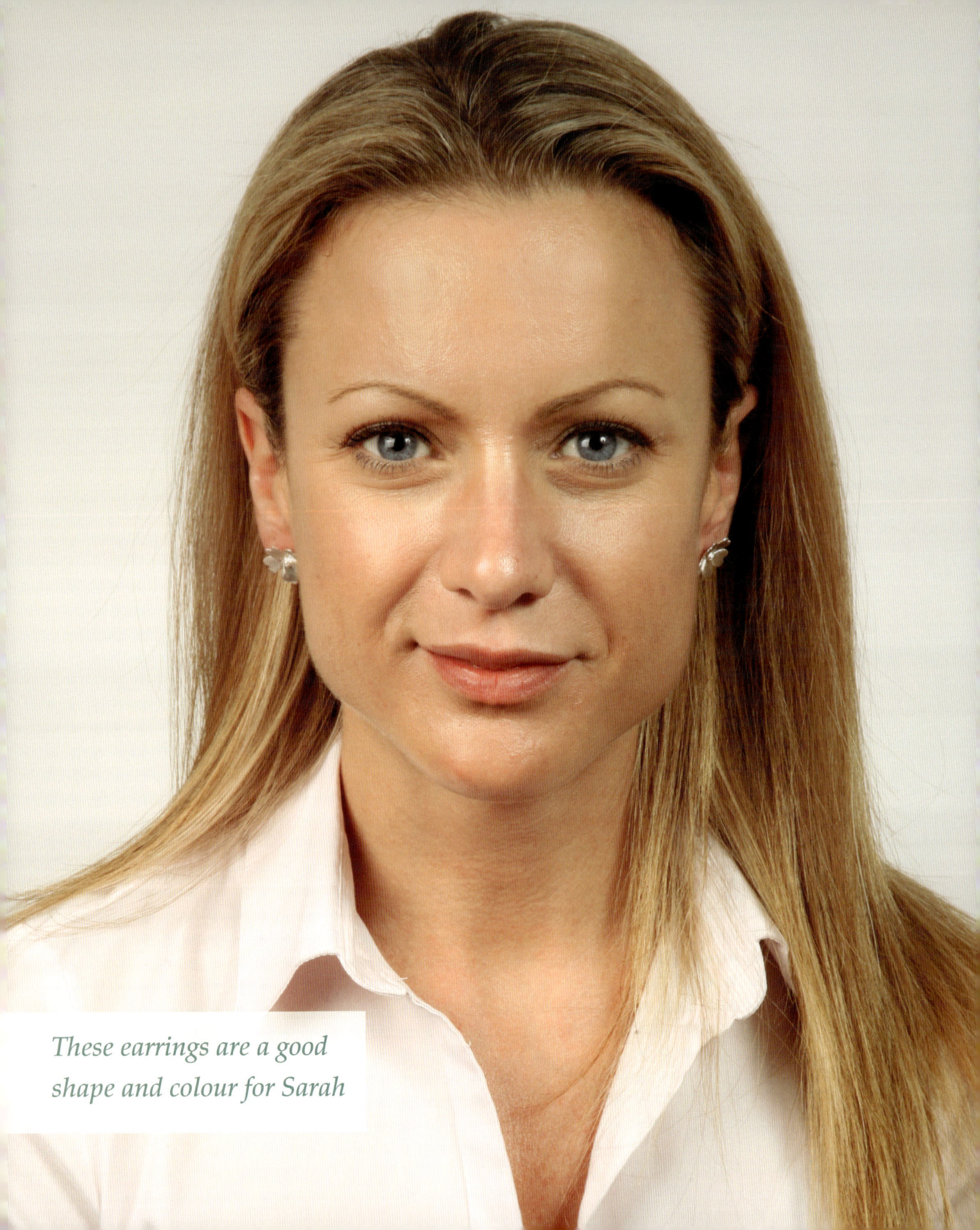

These earrings are a good shape and colour for Sarah

CHAPTER THREE: EARRINGS & FACE SHAPE

Sarah has an inverted triangle face shape but has a fairly square, angular jaw edge. Sarah therefore needs to avoid angular earrings and opt for rounded shapes instead. Stud earrings are good for Sarah.

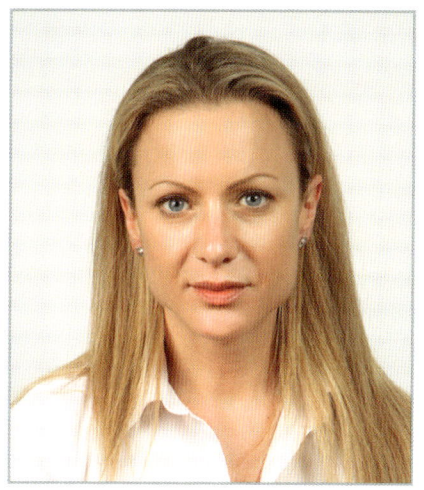

These are the correct colour and shape for her face. As long as her hair doesn't fall over her ears they are a good earring choice for her.

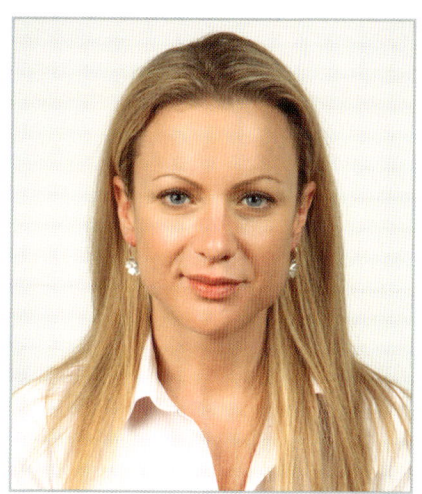

If Sarah wishes to wear dangly earrings she must choose either very short or very long earrings and avoid earrings that finish on the square edge of her jaw. These earrings are slightly too long; if they hung just below her ear lobe they would be more appropriate.

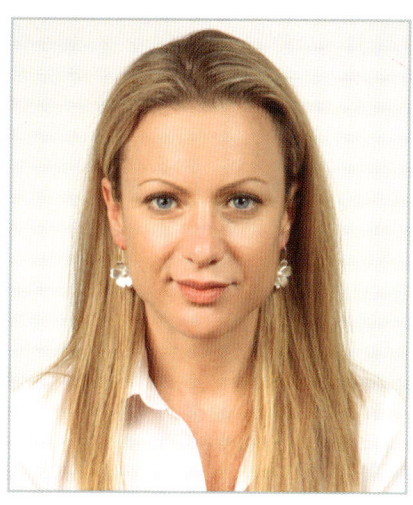

Note how these earrings, though a good colour for Sarah, widen her face and draw attention to the square edge of her jawline.

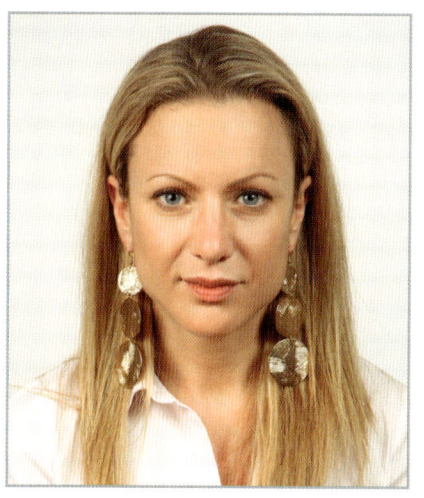

These earrings are the wrong colour for Sarah and much too big for her smaller frame. The earrings would work if they were silver hoops rather than solid discs and the bottom disc was removed. The earrings would then fall just below chin level. The round shapes mask the square edge to her jaw and would be suitable for an evening function. (Note how a drop of only one disc would exaggerate her square jaw.)

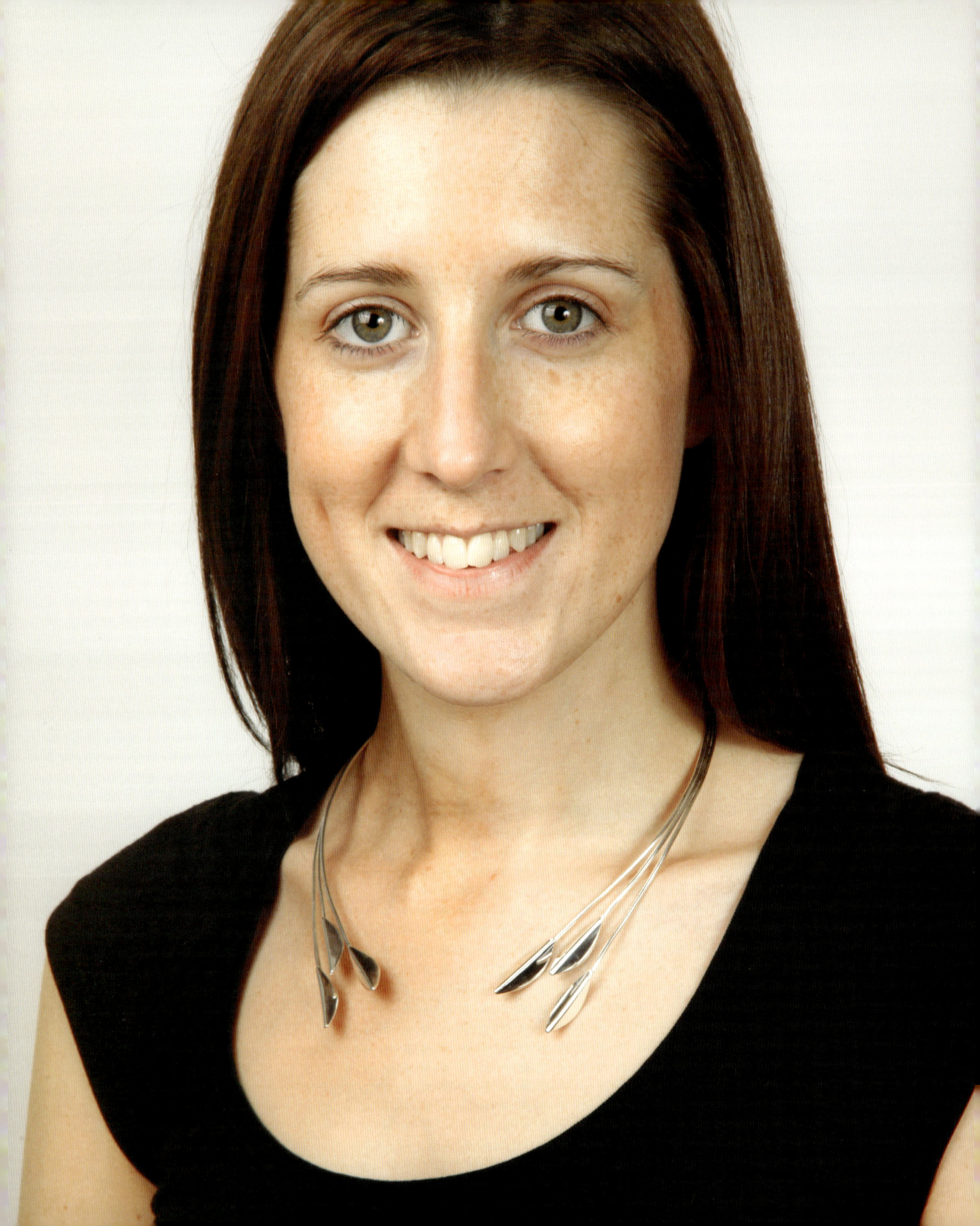

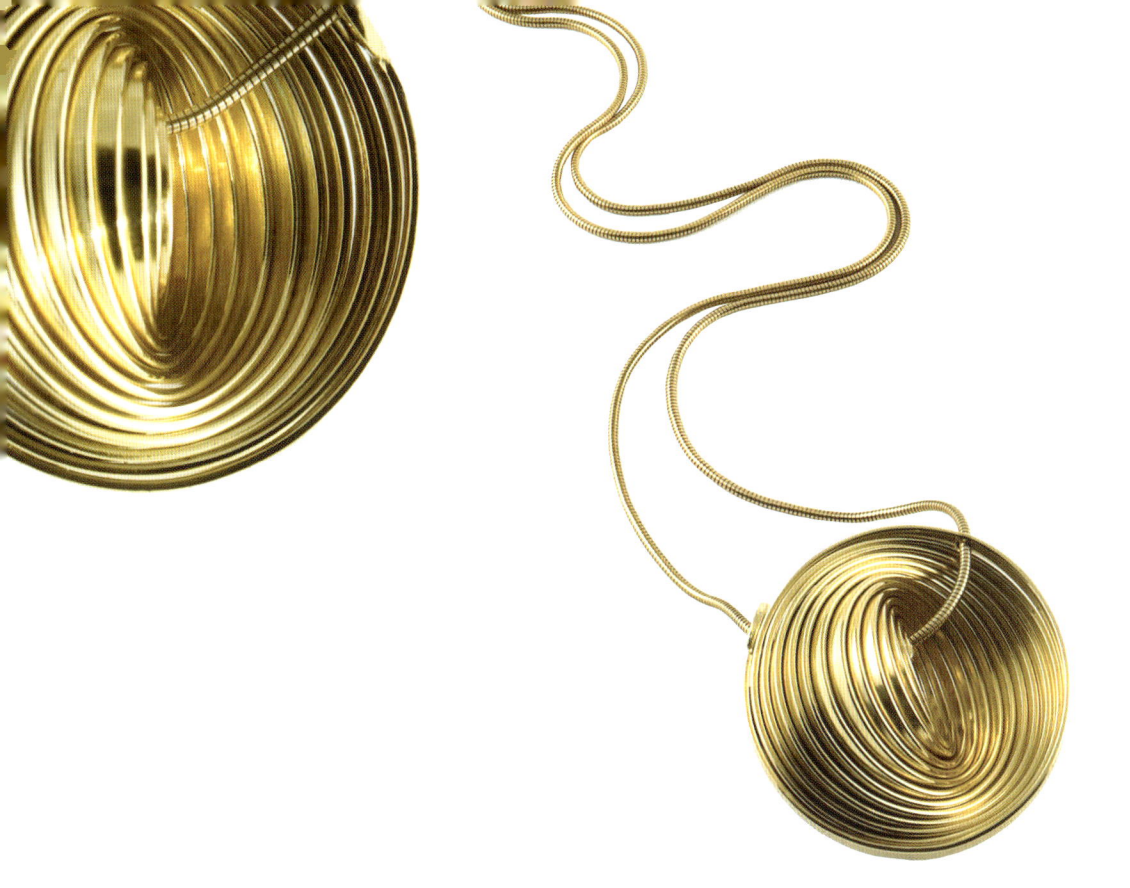

Chapter Four

Necklaces

Does This Look Good On Me?

Necklaces

Necklaces are one of the oldest forms of jewellery and can be made in a great many types of material. Most women have at least one necklace, and usually many more than one in their collection. In this section only the physical features of the necklace wearer are to be considered.

The perfect necklace:

- Should enhance your good features and disguise any flaws
- Take into account neck length and width
- Be appropriate for your build i.e. small and delicate for a small frame and chunkier for the larger frame
- Compliment the outfit to be worn
- Take into account the occasion for which it is to be worn

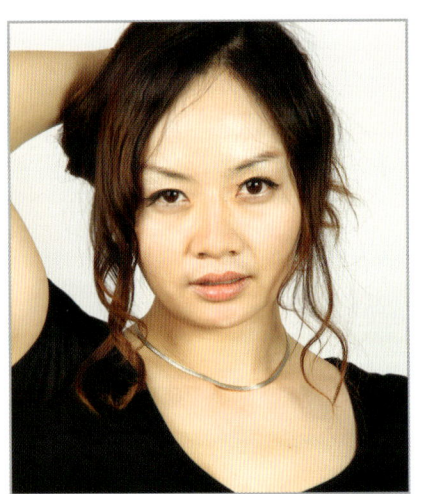 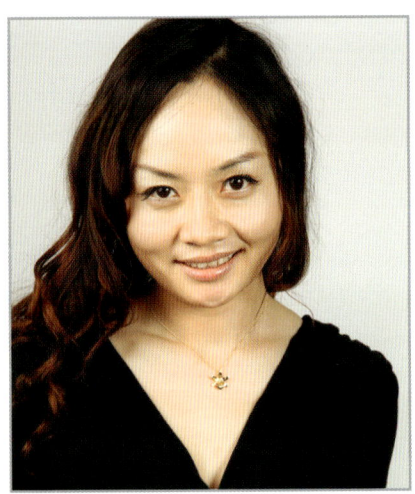 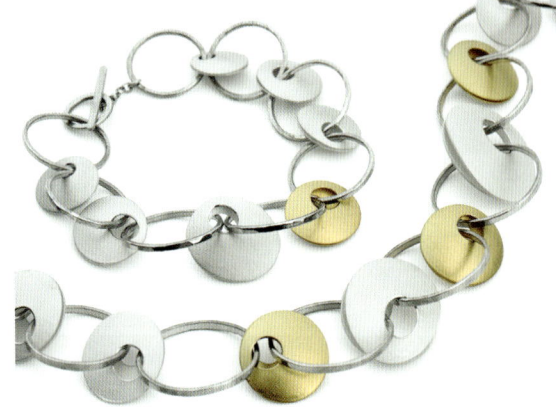

Evelyn likes fine, delicate necklaces. The first gold necklace (above left), although simple and delicate is a little short and makes her neck appear wider and shorter. The second pendant (above right) is better as it is very delicate and the chain is longer so it doesn't emphasise her neck. A chain that was slightly longer, allowing the pendant to hang 2 or 3 cm lower, would be ideal.

34

CHAPTER FOUR: NECKLACES

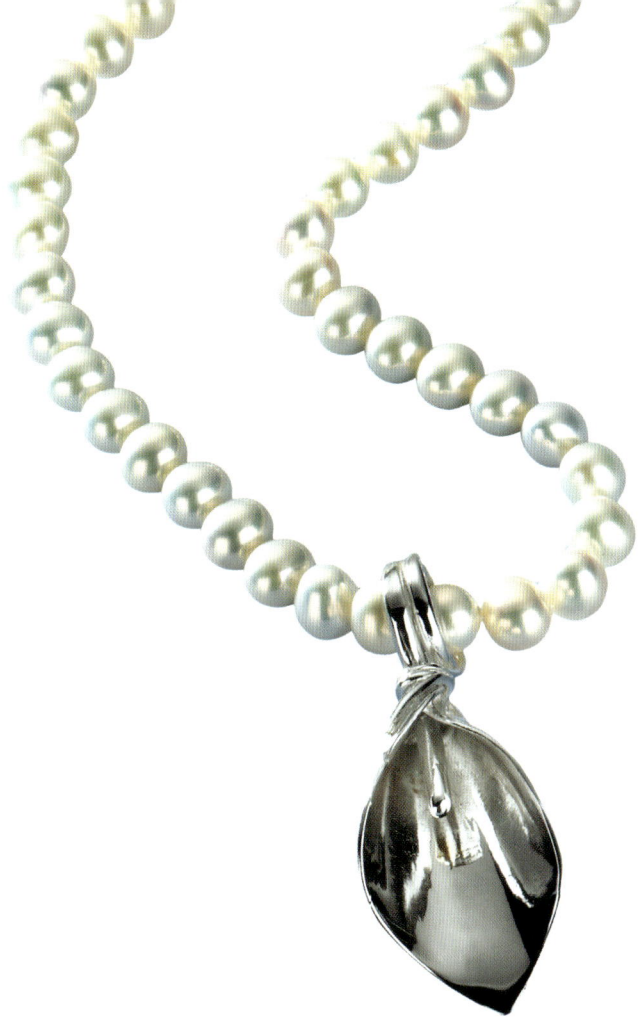

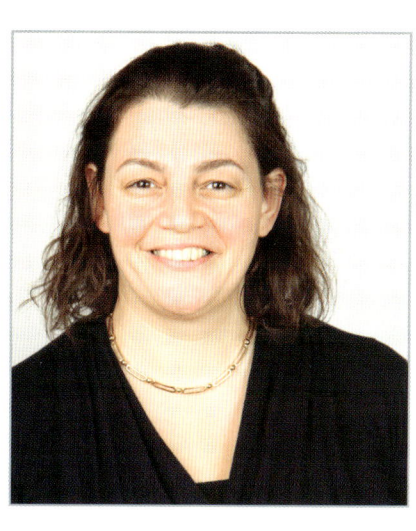

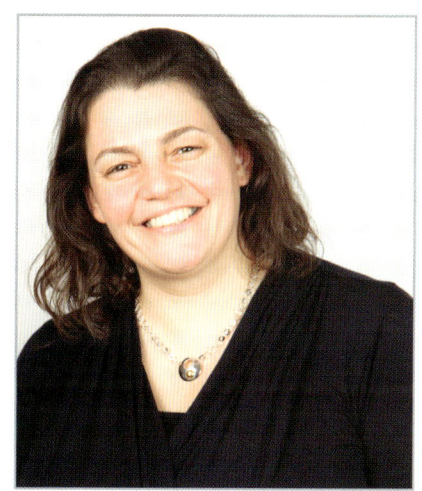

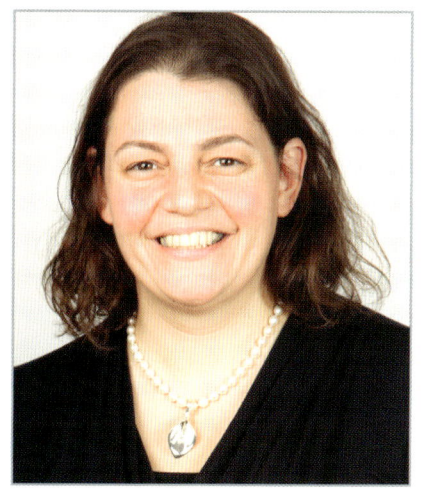

Observe the images of Helena to the right.

The top photograph shows Helena in a short, gold, choker style necklace. This necklace is not the ideal metal colour for Helena, as she suits silver better. It is also too short for her neck size. Note how this necklace draws attention to her neck, making it appear wider.

The centre photograph shows Helena wearing a silver pendant on a heavier silver chain. The colour, length and style of the chain is much better for Helena, however the shape of the pendant emphasises the roundness of her face.

The Arum Lily Pendant in the bottom photograph is a much better shape for Helena. The elongated lily does not mimic her round face. The pendant hangs midway between her neck and bust, thereby not emphasizing either of these areas. The white pearls compliment Helena's colouring and are classical, therefore versatile. Should Helena wish to change the look of this pendant is is easy to slip the pendant off the pearls and put it onto another string of coloured beads or a heavy silver chain.

Does This Look Good On Me?

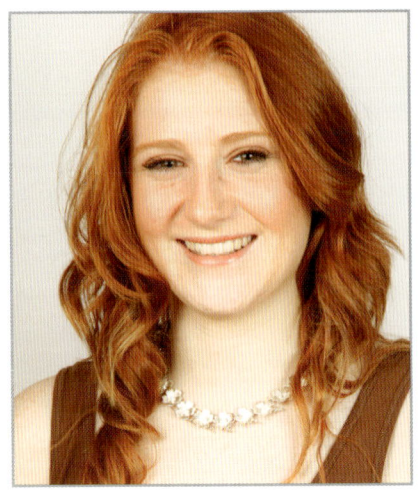
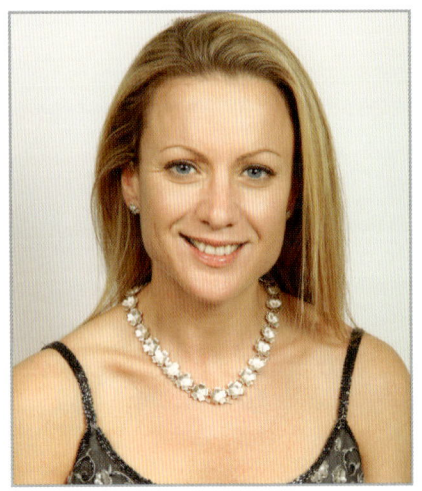
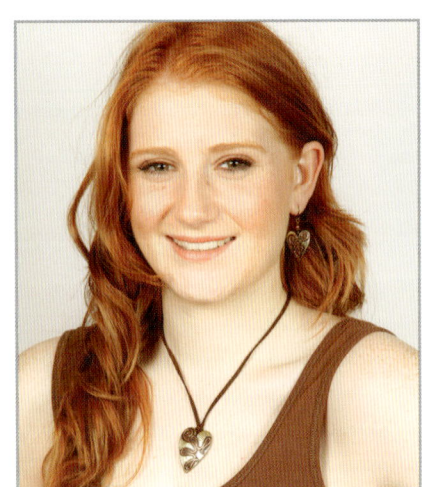

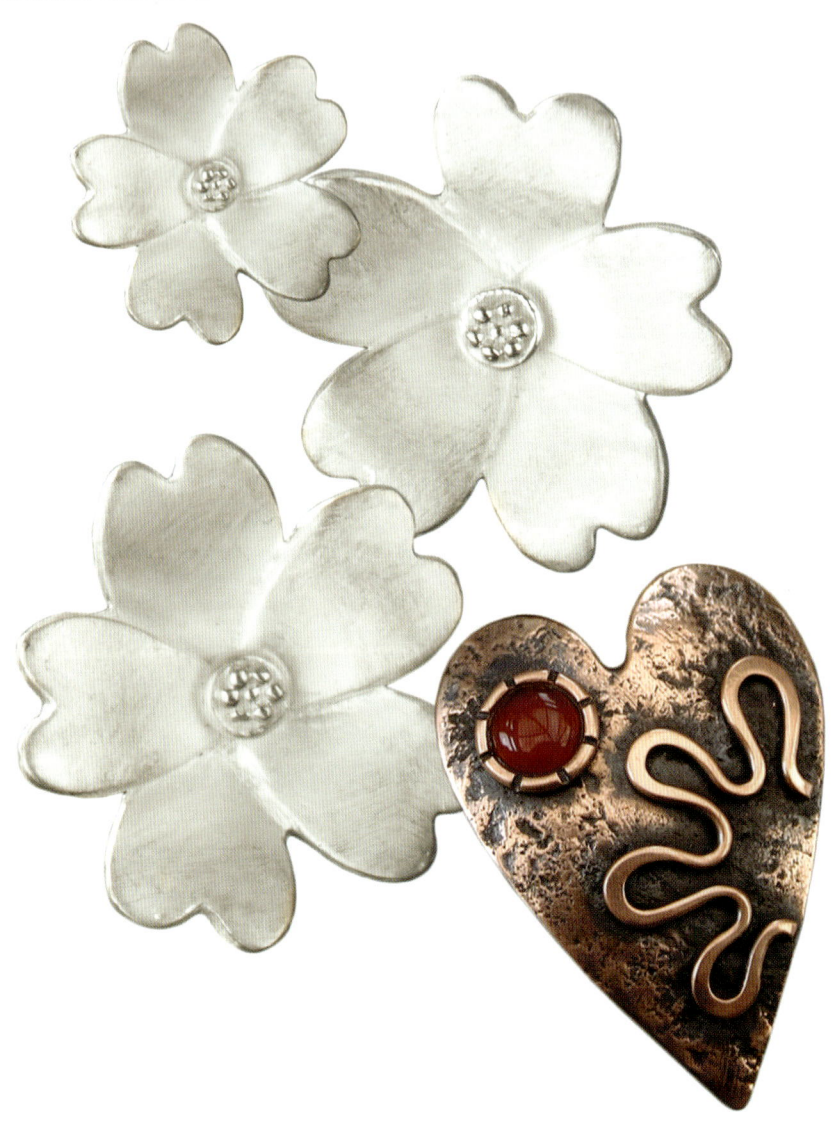

Look at the primrose necklace being worn by Danielle and Sarah above.

Both girls are the right size and shape for the necklace, but it looks amazing on Sarah and uninspiring on Danielle. Why?

Danielle's vibrant red hair and pale skin is not complimented by silver, she needs gold or copper-coloured metals.

Sarah's blonde hair, blue eyes and warmer skin tone is complimented by silver. Danielle is wearing a very casual vest top so the style of necklace doesn't quite match either her outfit or the casual everyday occasion.

Danielle looks so much better in the copper and brass pendant and earrings, which are more appropriate for her outfit and the occasion.

Sarah wanted a necklace to compliment her silver and grey cocktail dress to attend an evening drinks party. Note how the matt silver primroses of the necklace and earrings compliment those on her dress to produce an elegant, sophisticated look, suitable for the occasion.

CHAPTER FOUR: NECKLACES

Beverley loves her jewellery and wears a great variety of different styles from several different designer/makers. She is particularly drawn to original pieces with interesting colour and stones. Both the white pearls and the blue apatite with 18ct gold necklaces are a good length for Beverley, focusing the eye midway between the neck and the bust. The white pearls give a sophisticated, elegant look and compliment her skin tone. The disc-shaped pearls offer a contemporary twist on the conventional string of pearls, appealing to Beverley's passion for different jewellery. The 18ct gold orchid provides a more dramatic, striking look especially when worn with the blue apatite, which perfectly compliments the blue of Beverley's eyes. This necklace will get her noticed, especially if she is wearing complimentary blue/turquoise clothing.

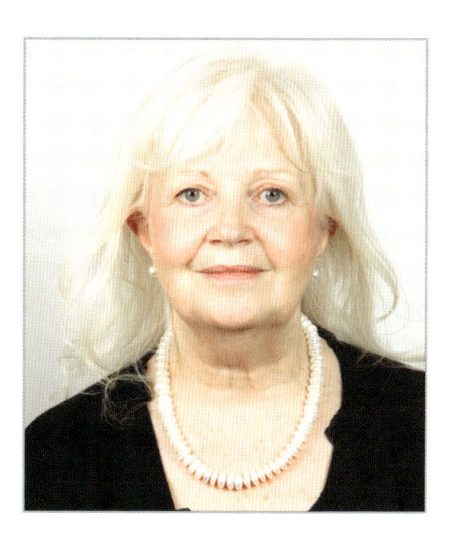

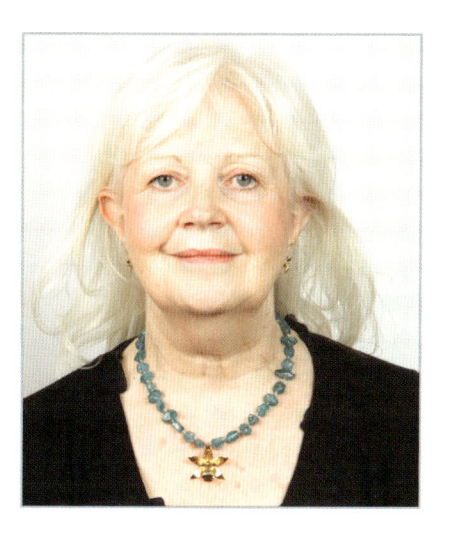

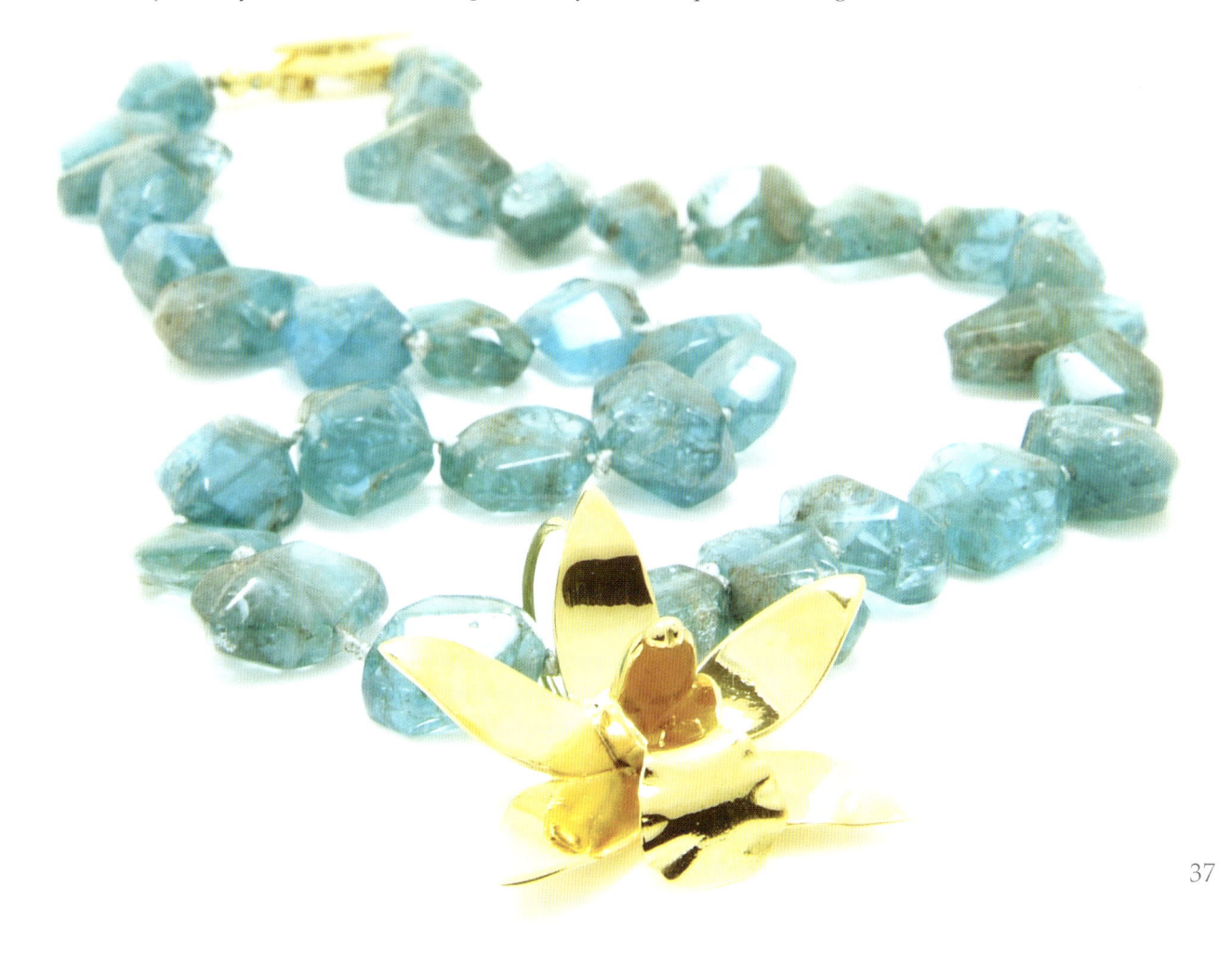

37

Does This Look Good On Me?

Evelyn is a fashion designer so image and fashion accessories are particularly important to her.

All three photos show dramatic statement piece necklaces.

The silver orchid on the labradorite (bottom right) is an attractive necklace, but the flower is slightly too large for Evelyn's build.

The colour of the beads and silver of the orchid are not ideal for Evelyn's skin tone.

The 18ct gold orchid on faceted rubies (top right) works better than the silver version as the gold suits her colouring.

The handcarved jade pendant (below) is probably the more appropriate statement necklace for Evelyn, as the green stone compliments her skin tone and the elongated pendant shape balances the roundness of her face.

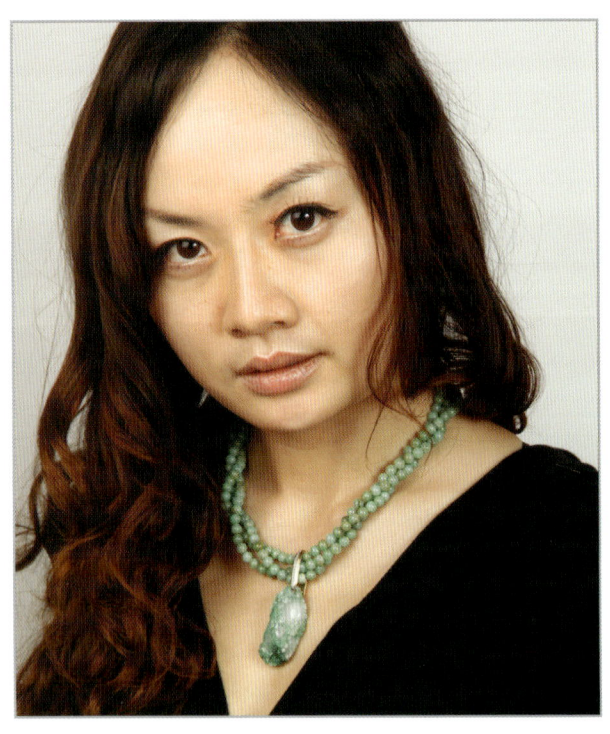

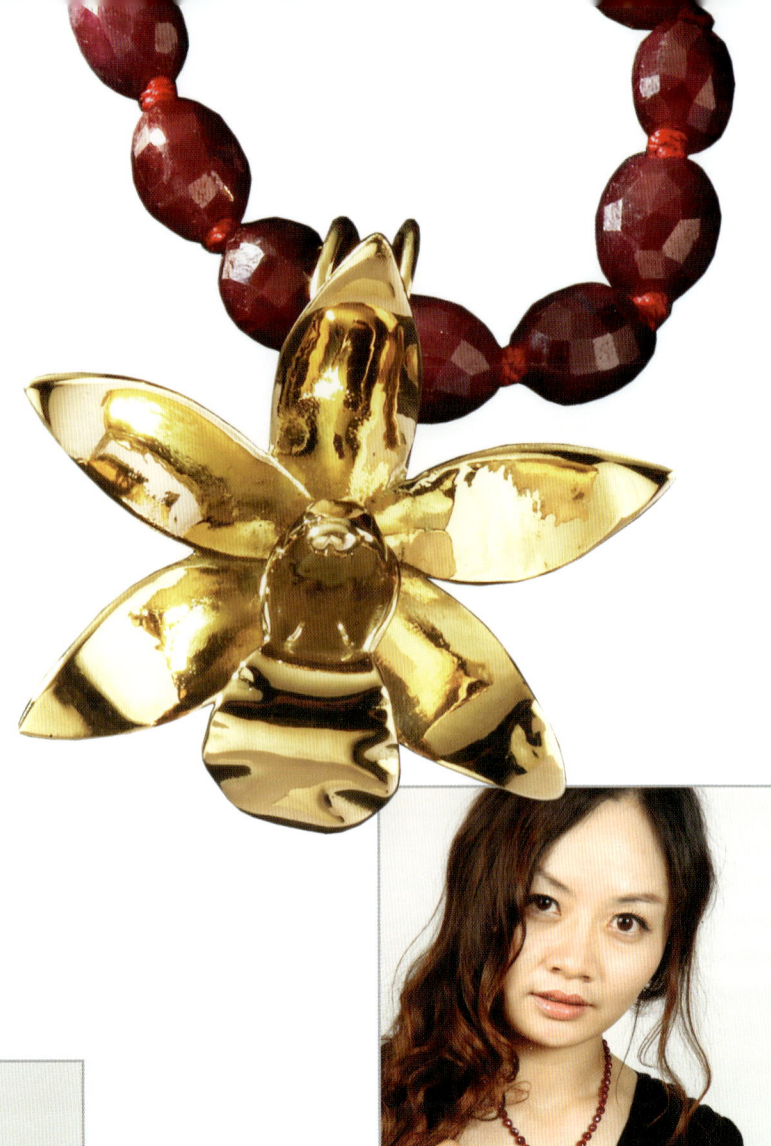

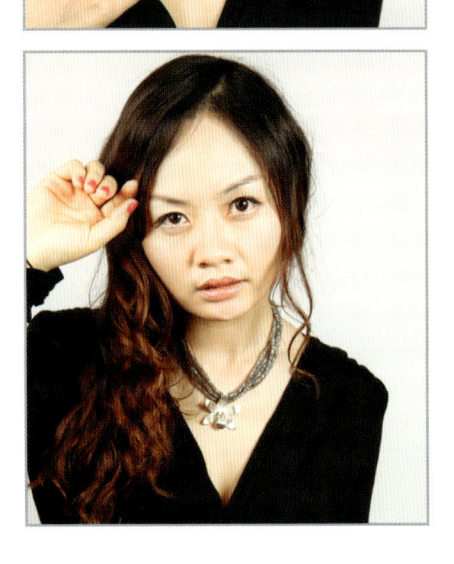

CHAPTER FOUR: NECKLACES

This 18ct gold necklace, chalcedony rose stone set with diamonds, looks good on Jade the gold compliments her skin tone, the roundness of the pendant balances her oblong face shape and the neutral colours in the stones make this a very versatile piece of jewellery, suitable for a range of occasions.

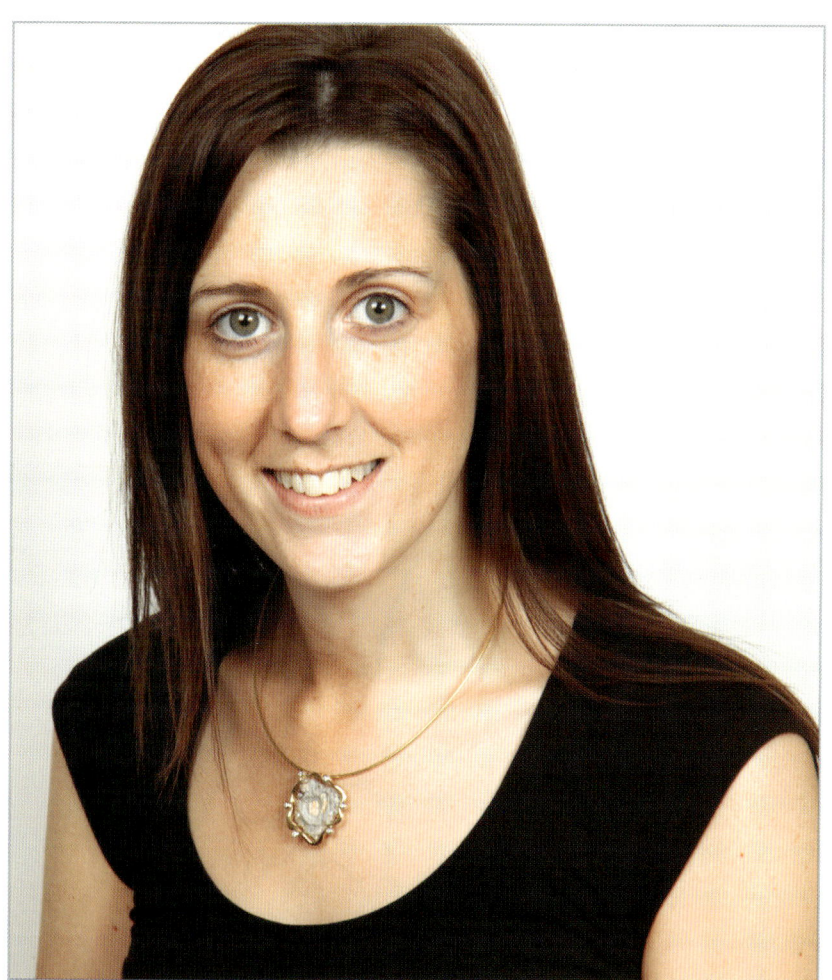

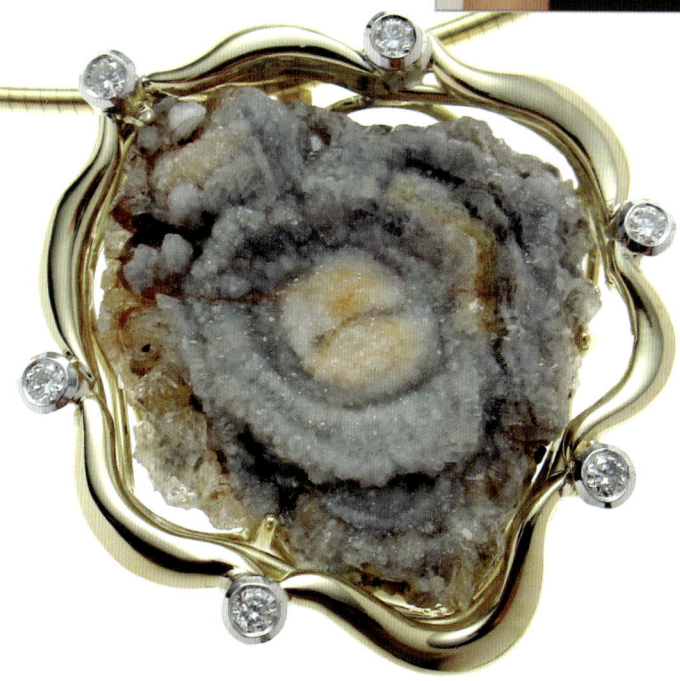

Silver cuff by KFD Jewellery

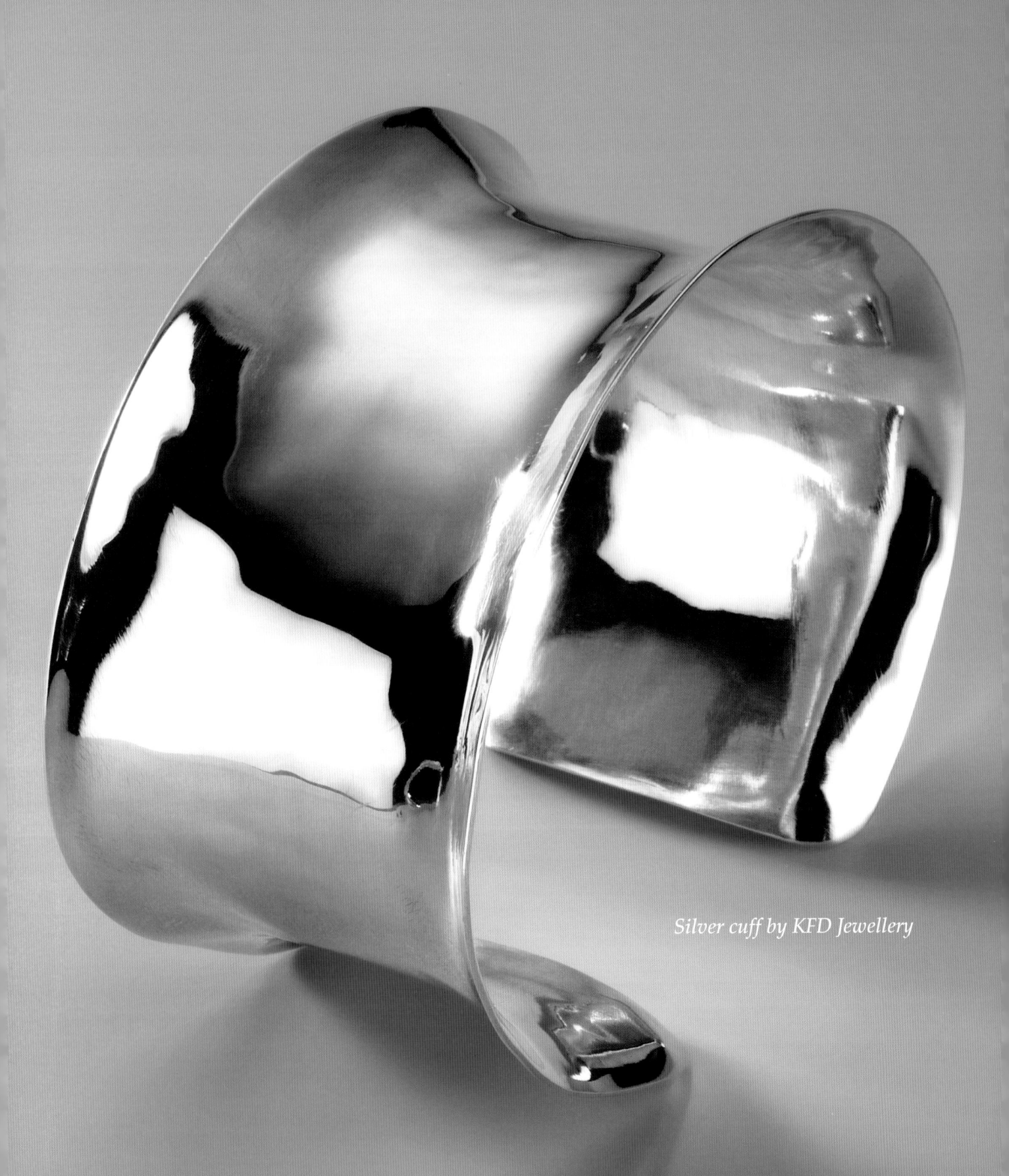

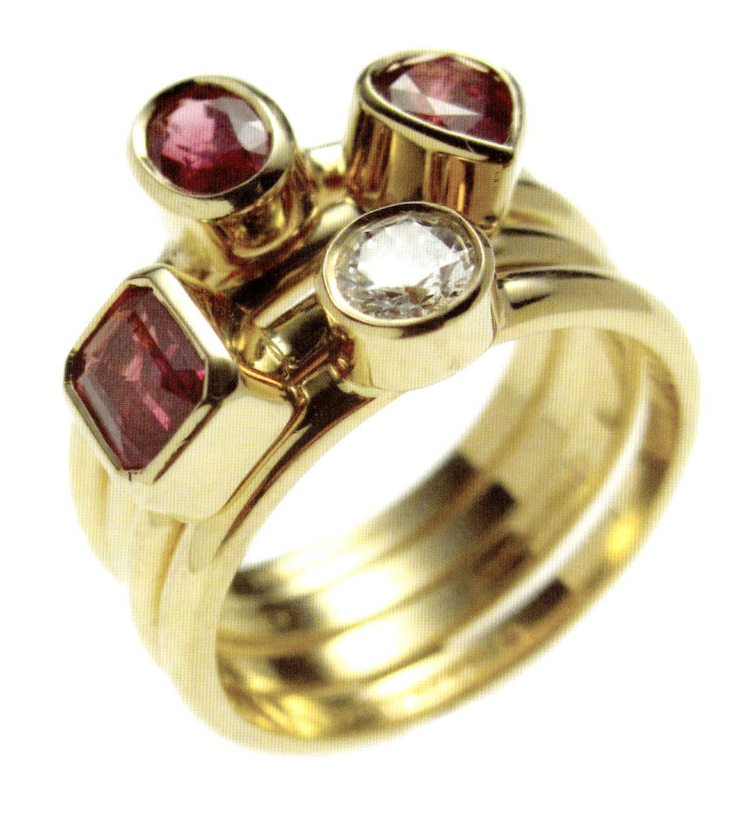

Chapter Five

Hand & Wrist

Bracelets & bangles

Bangles, bracelets and cuffs are very fashionable jewellery items. If a necklace is not suitable for your outfit, it may well be the case that a carefully chosen bracelet can be the perfect accessory to finish your look. The size of your hand and your wrist is an important consideration when choosing a bracelet. If your hands are large and wrist broad then a fine delicate bangle will look too small whereas a chunky statement bracelet is more appropriate. A small hand and narrow wrist looks good with a delicate bracelet and is over powered by a large, chunky bracelet. This is clearly demonstrated in the illustrations on the facing page.

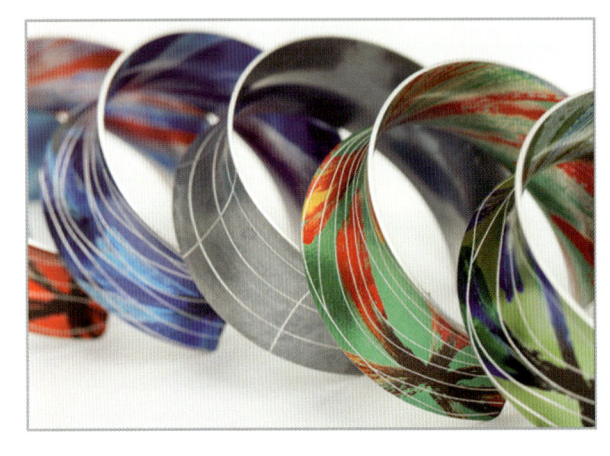

Once you have decided on the relative size of the bracelet, consider how the colour of the bracelet works with your skin tone.

Looking at the photographs on the right, the images on the left hand side look good with the silver, but note how the hands on the right hand side do not.

Compare these with the diagrams below where the size of bracelet is correct for the hand, but the metal has been changed to gold.

This comparison was more obvious when the whole person was viewed with the bracelet.

The hand on the left belongs to Helena – a silver person. The hand on the right is Evelyn's – a gold person.

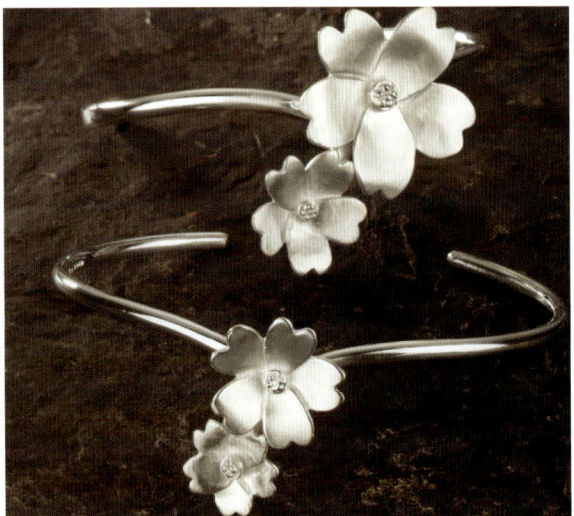

The bracelet illustrated left is the one worn by Helena and Evelyn (centre photos, right). It is from the Primose collection by KFD Jewllery

Chapter Five: Hand & Wrist

Helena's hand

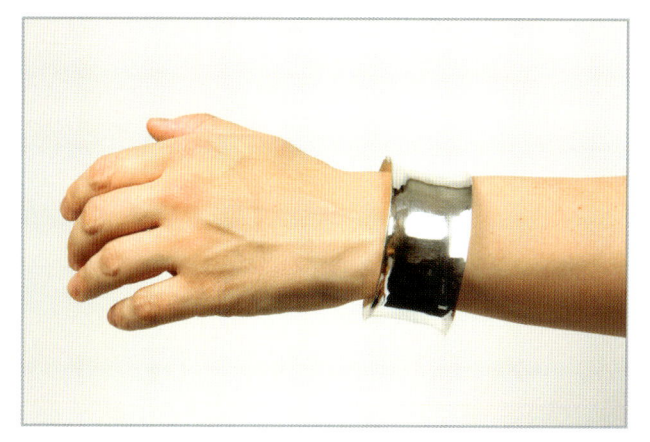

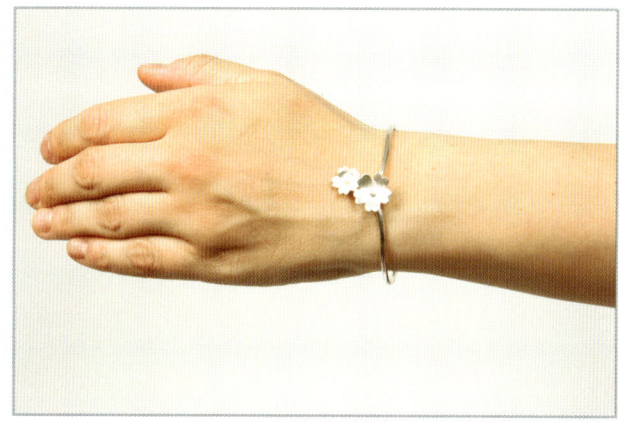

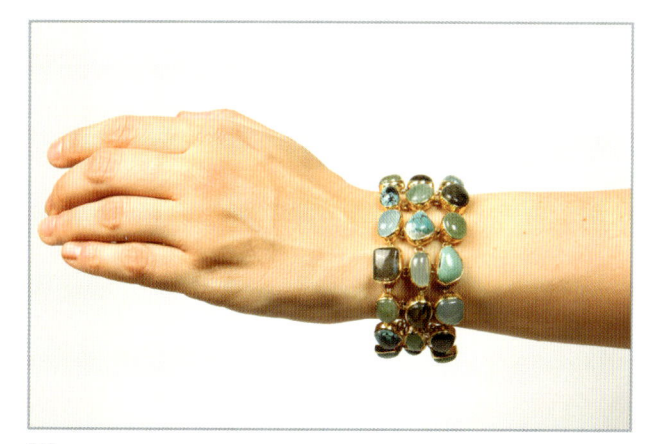

Evelyn's hand

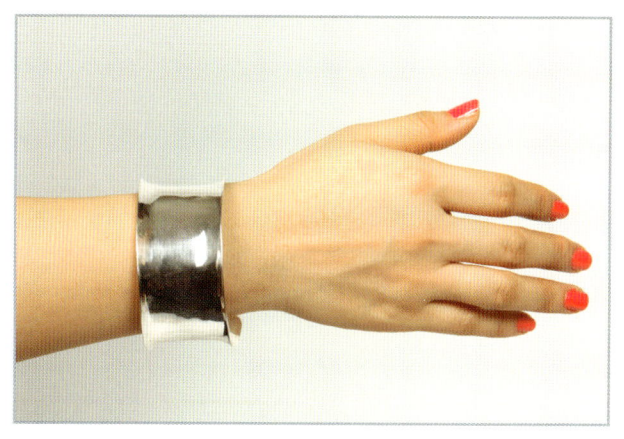

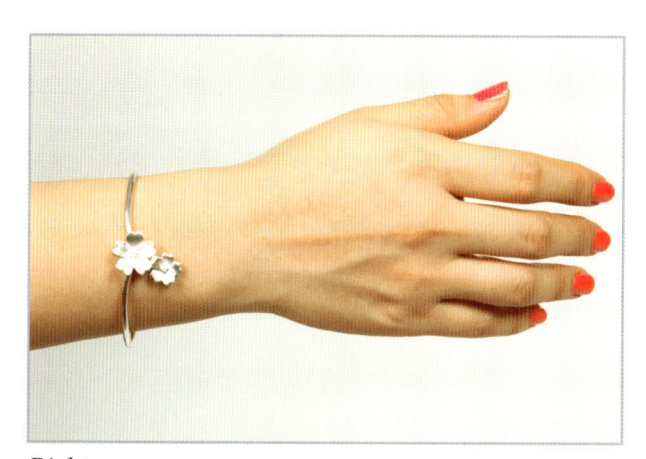

Right

Wrong

Wrong

Right

Wrong

Right

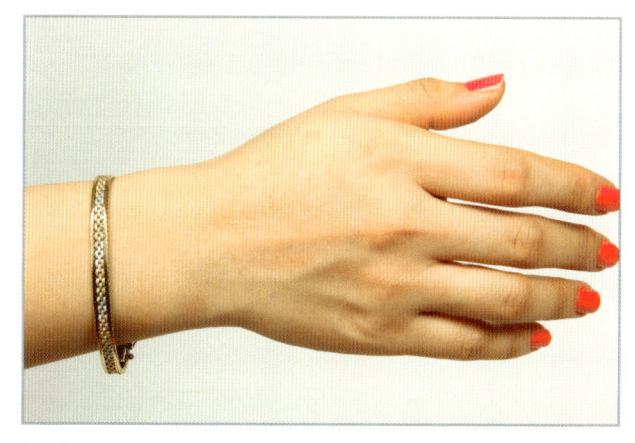

43

Does This Look Good On Me?

Rings

A ring is a piece of jewellery which most women have. Some women have rings that they wear constantly, such as a wedding band, whilst other rings are changed according to the occasion or to suit one's outfit. Occasion and personal choice will be discussed in a later chapter, for now we will consider hand size.

The perfect ring hand has long slender fingers and well groomed nails. If you are fortunate to have hands such as these then you can wear most types of ring. If your fingers are short relative to the size of your hand then, no matter if your hand is slim or plump, you are limited in the design of ring that will look good on your hand. As with all jewellery, if you are petite then smaller, more delicate rings are appropriate; big rings will look clumpy on your hand. If you have large hands, chunkier rings will look better.

Evelyn's hand is 3½ cm shorter but her fingers are almost as long as Sarah's. Note how Evelyn's hands look more elegant because she has relatively long fingers compared to the size of her palm. Compare Sarah's hand in the four band width to Evelyn's hand in the same four bands. Although three bands may have been better for Evelyn, she could wear all four bands of these stackable rings even though she has very small hands.

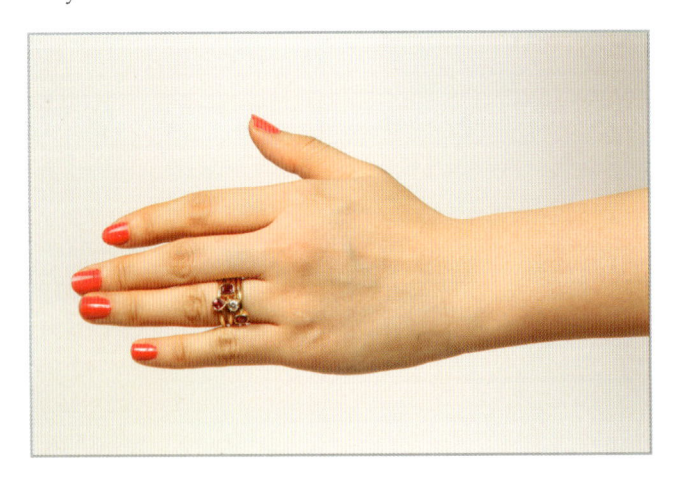

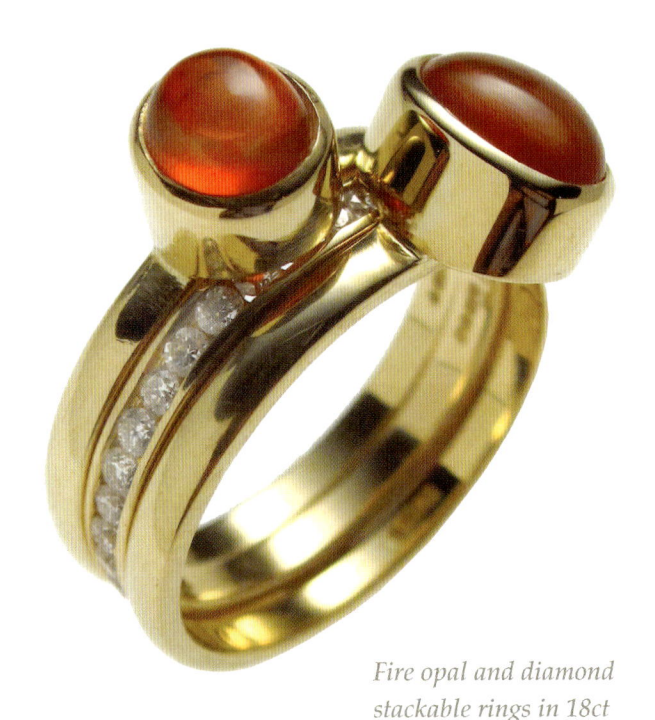

Fire opal and diamond stackable rings in 18ct gold by Susan Vedadi

CHAPTER FIVE: HAND & WRIST

Sarah's hand

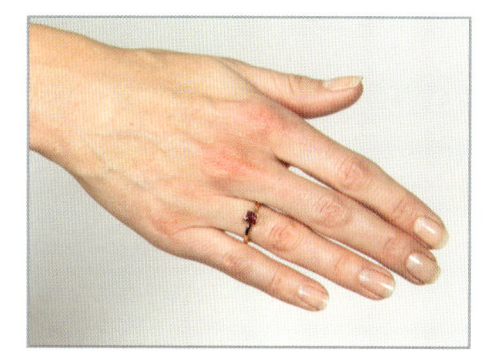

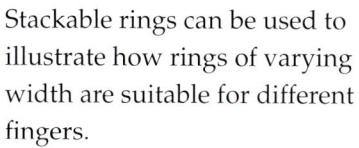

Danielle's hand

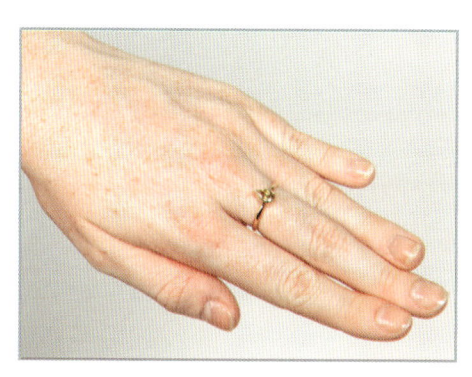

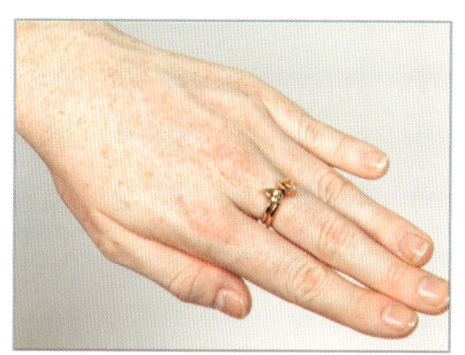

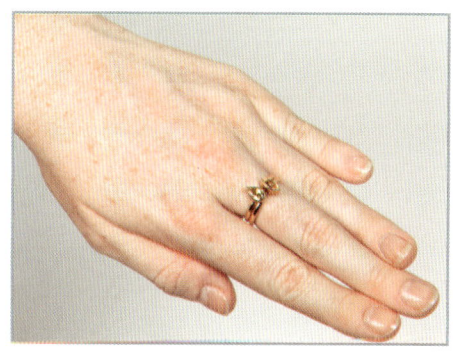

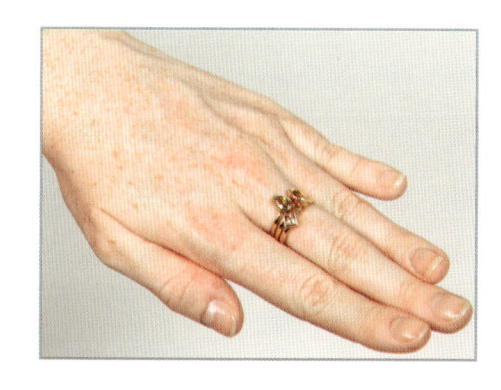

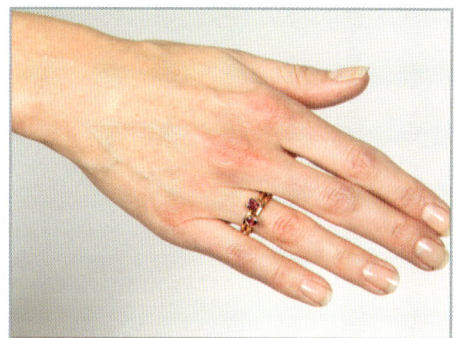

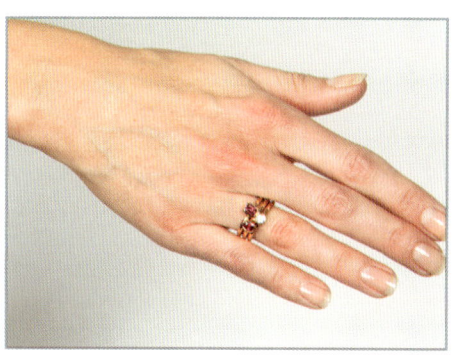

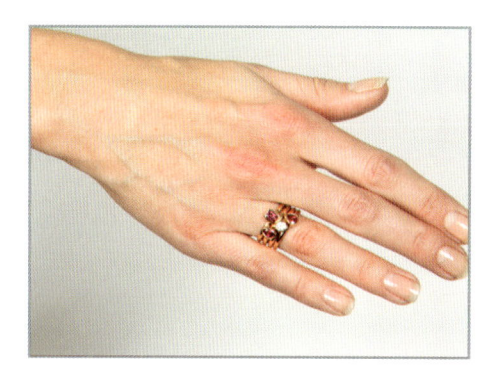

Stackable rings can be used to illustrate how rings of varying width are suitable for different fingers.

Sarah's hand is only very slightly longer than Danielle's, but Danielle's fingers are longer and her palm size smaller than Sarah's.

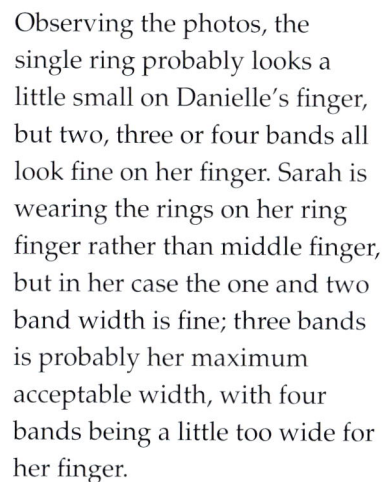

Observing the photos, the single ring probably looks a little small on Danielle's finger, but two, three or four bands all look fine on her finger. Sarah is wearing the rings on her ring finger rather than middle finger, but in her case the one and two band width is fine; three bands is probably her maximum acceptable width, with four bands being a little too wide for her finger.

This illustrates that a longer finger length relative to palm size allows wider ring bands to be worn.

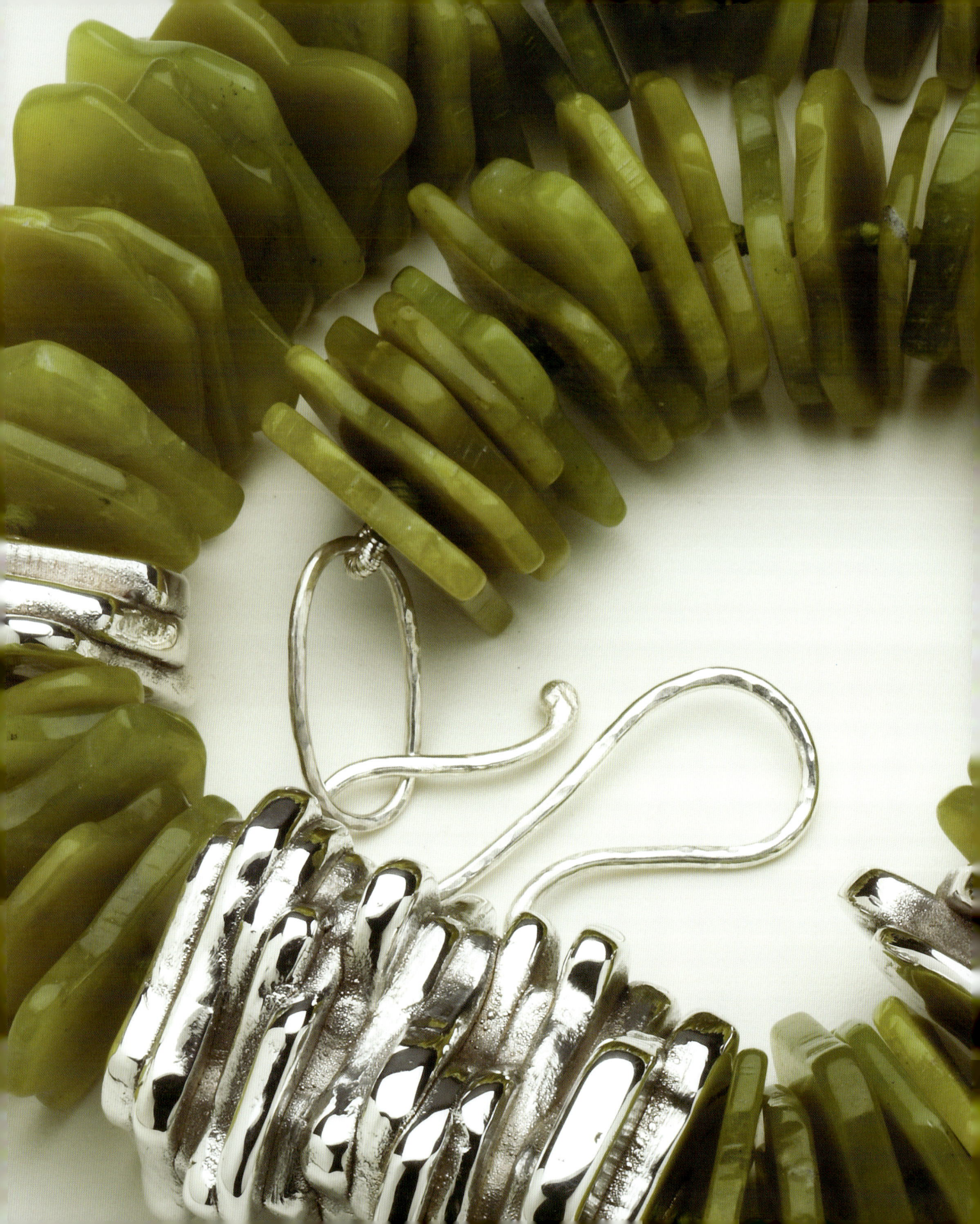

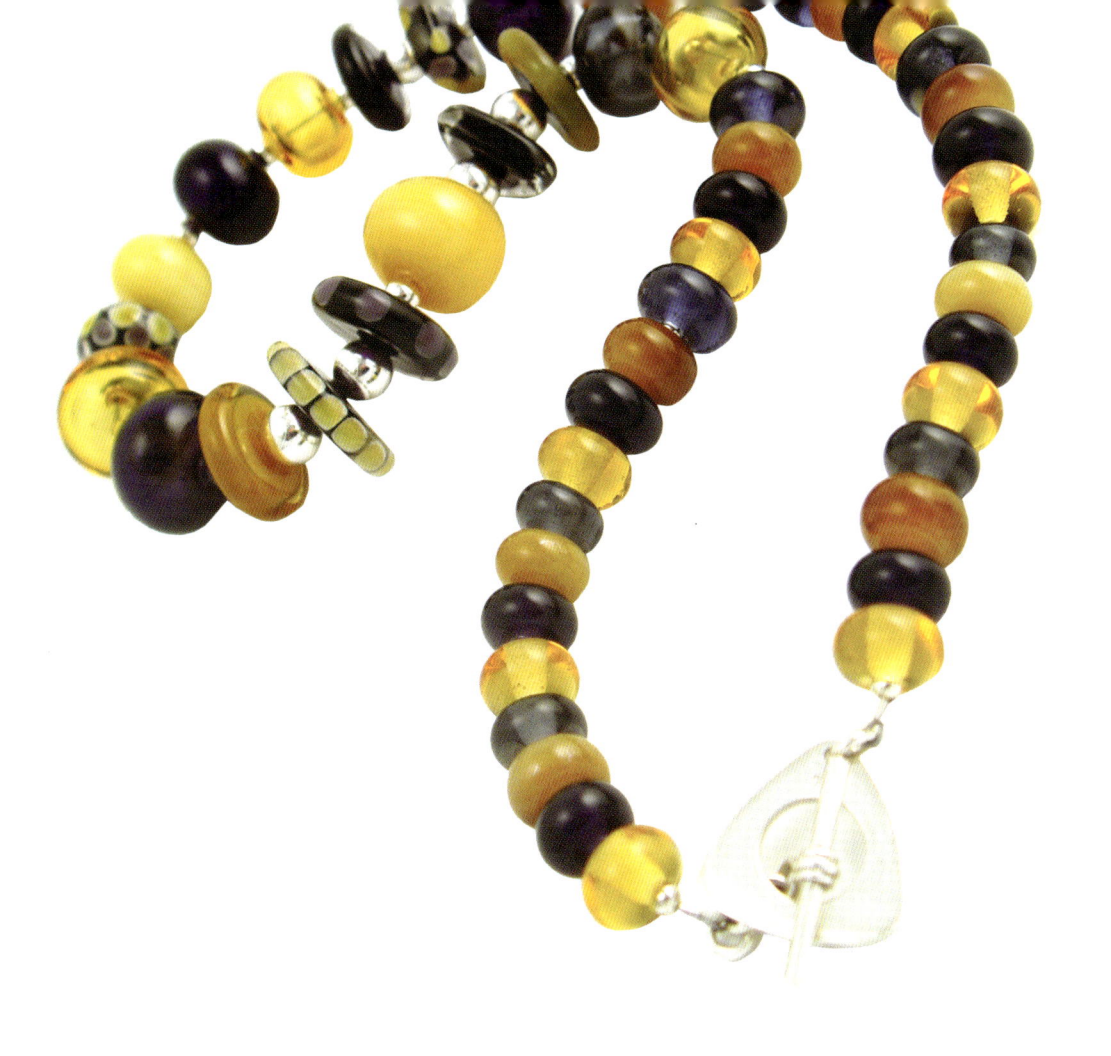

Chapter Six

Colour

Colour and jewellery

Colour is a part of our everyday life. Colour can evoke emotion, influence our behavior and determine whether or not we want to eat a certain food. The colours we wear influence how we feel and how others perceive us.

The meaning of the colours you wear

There has been considerable research and much written about the meaning of colour, but here is a brief summary of the main points:

Red: Confidence, action, courage, vitality, but also danger and anger.

Orange: Vitality, endurance, increased creativity.

Brown: Earth, order and convention, but also a repressed character.

Yellow: Happiness, good health, vitality, creative and intellectual clarity.

Green: The symbol of nature. Represents restful tranquility. Is the colour of balance and harmony.

Blue: Calmness, inspiration, sincerity, spirituality, serenity, but also coldness.

Purple: The colour of royalty, good judgment, spiritual fulfillment and magic and mystery.

White: Purity and mental clarity.

Black: Formality, sophistication, death.

Grey: Responsible, conservative practicality.

Pink: Love, beauty, femininity, caring, protection against violence.

Coloured jewellery

Coloured jewellery can be used to harmonise with your natural colouring, or to introduce contrast and drama into your outfit. There is a wealth of coloured jewellery on the market from both designer makers and the High Street, with prices to suit all budgets. Here are a few examples of techniques used to produce coloured jewellery from a selection of designers currently living and working in the UK.

CHAPTER SIX: COLOUR

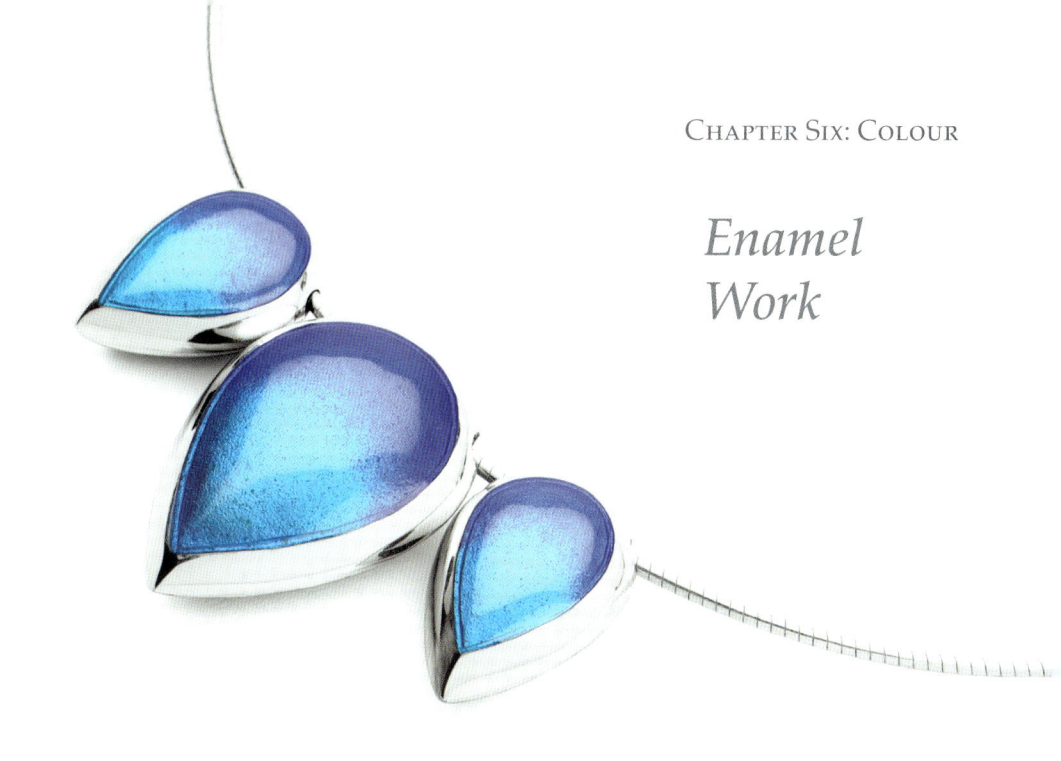

Enamel Work

Enamelling is a labour-intensive technique used by jewellers to apply colour to metals such as silver, gold, copper and steel. Essentially enamel is a finely ground glass which, when fired in a furnace at high temperatures, produces a layer of colour over the metal.

There are three different types of enamel, translucent, opaque and opalescent. Translucent enamels allow the background metal to be seen. Jewellers may use hand or machine engraving techniques to pattern the metal before applying the enamel.

Opaque enamels obscure the metal background. Opalescent enamels are slightly milky is appearance.

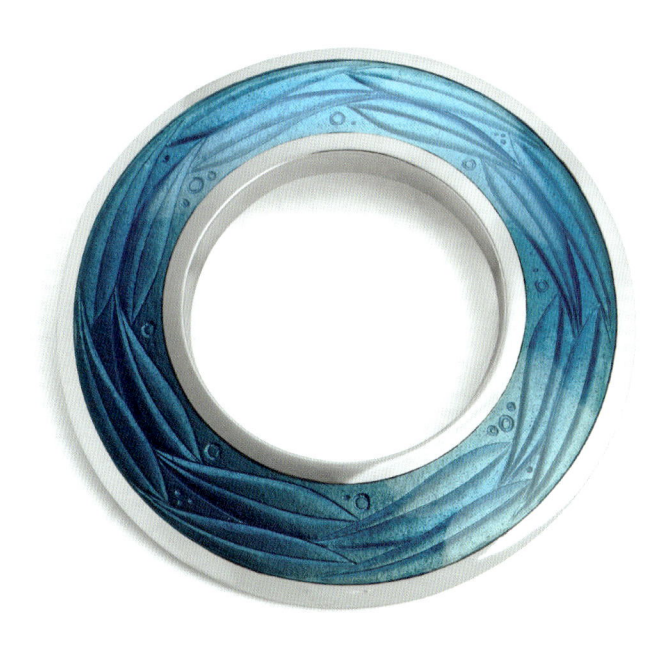

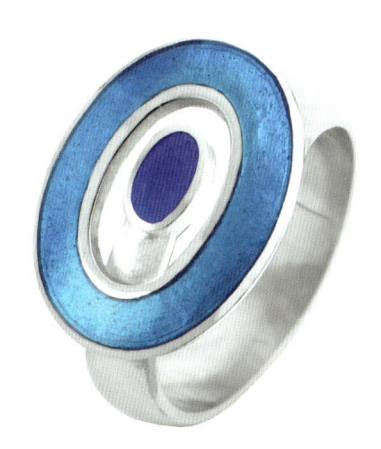

Rachel Gogerly is a jeweller and silversmith who often makes use of translucent enamels in her designs.

Coloured stones

Semi-precious and precious stones have been used throughout history to add colour to jewellery. The inclusion of precious stones not only adds colour, but also signifies opulence and wealth. The sparkle induced by faceted stones adds to the desirability of the stones, making them highly prized. Precious stones are not always within the reach of all consumers. Consequently there is a huge industry in the production of simulated 'precious' stones to make costume jewellery.

Susan Vedadi has a workshop in the heart of the Jewellery Quarter in Birmingham. Susan designs and makes one-off pieces of jewellery in gold with both precious and semi-precious stones. The stones are central to Susan's designs. Each piece of jewellery is totally unique and designed to enhance the natural beauty of the stone.

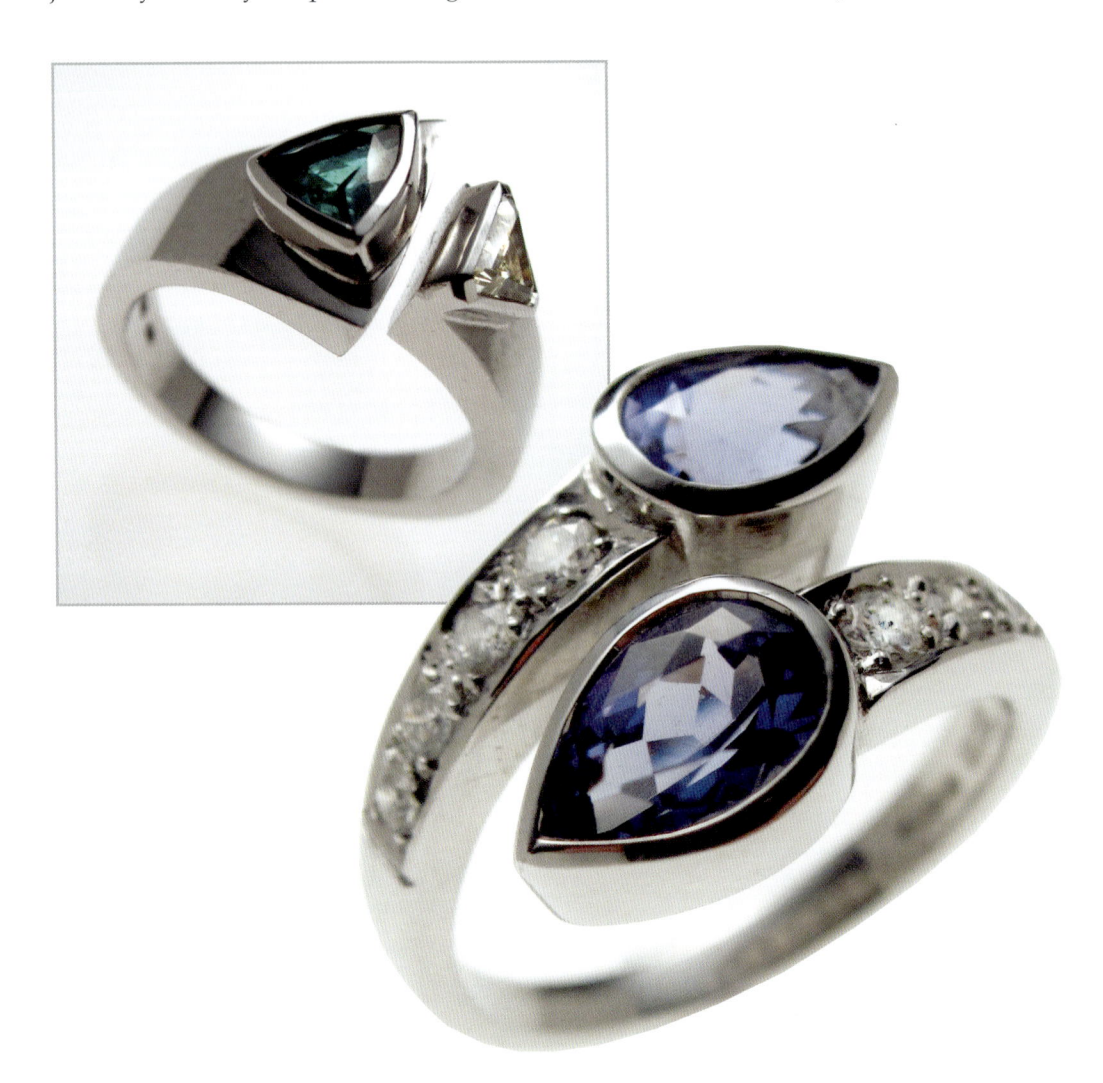

Top: Colombian emerald and yellow diamond in white gold

Bottom: Tanzanite and diamond in white gold

Both by Susan Vedadi

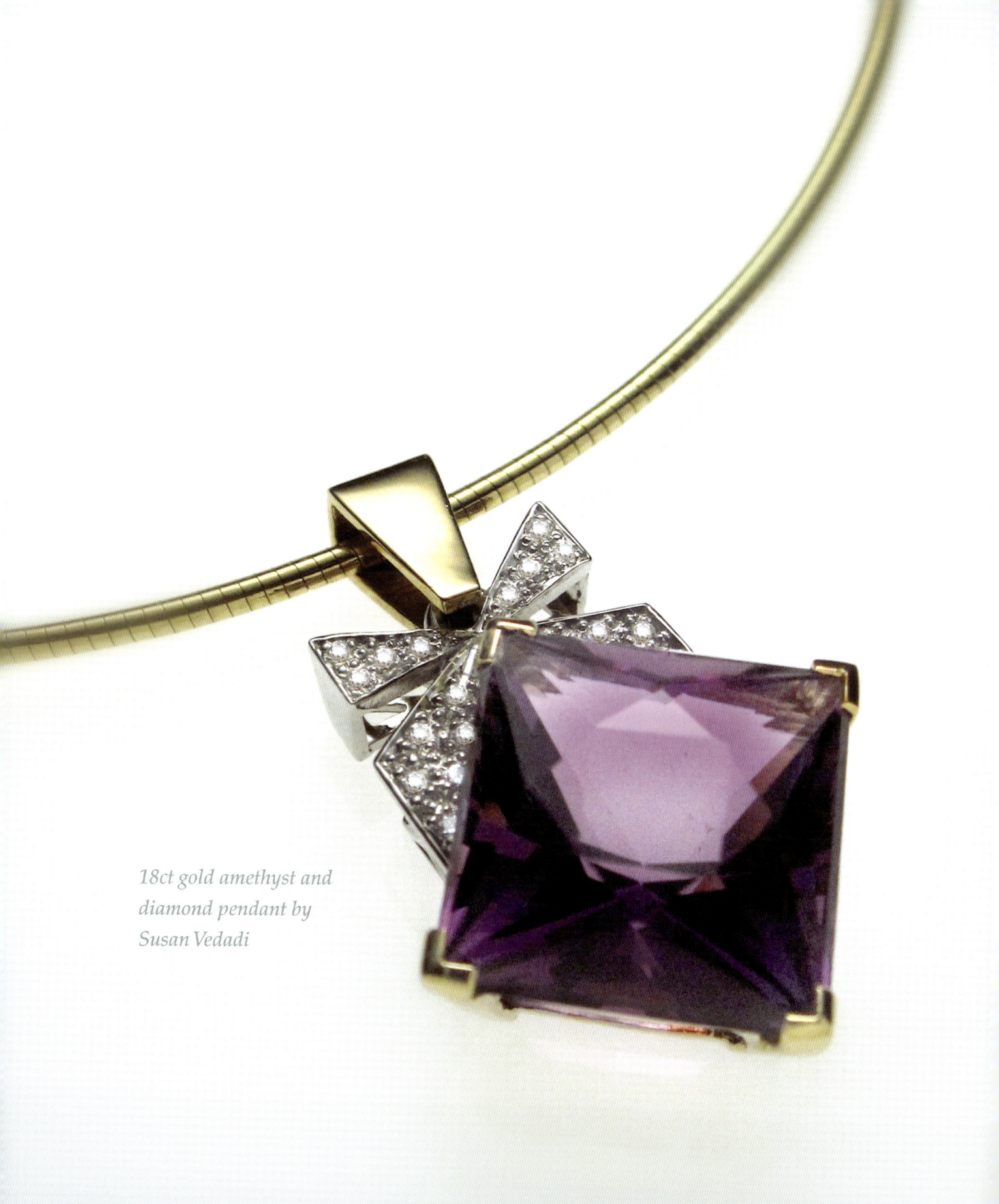

*18ct gold amethyst and
diamond pendant by
Susan Vedadi*

Precious & semi-precious stone beads

The exciting colours, patterns and textures found in semi–precious stones make them a fabulous material for jewellery making. Semi-precious beads exist in a vast range of shapes and sizes and can be faceted, rough cut or polished.

Beads can be used to change the look of a statement pendant. The 18ct gold Orchid pendant *(KFD Jewellery)* looks very different worn with the faceted rubies as opposed to the rough cut appatite stone beads. As the pendant is removable it could be worn with other beads or pearls to give a different 'feel' to the statement necklace.

CHAPTER SIX: COLOUR

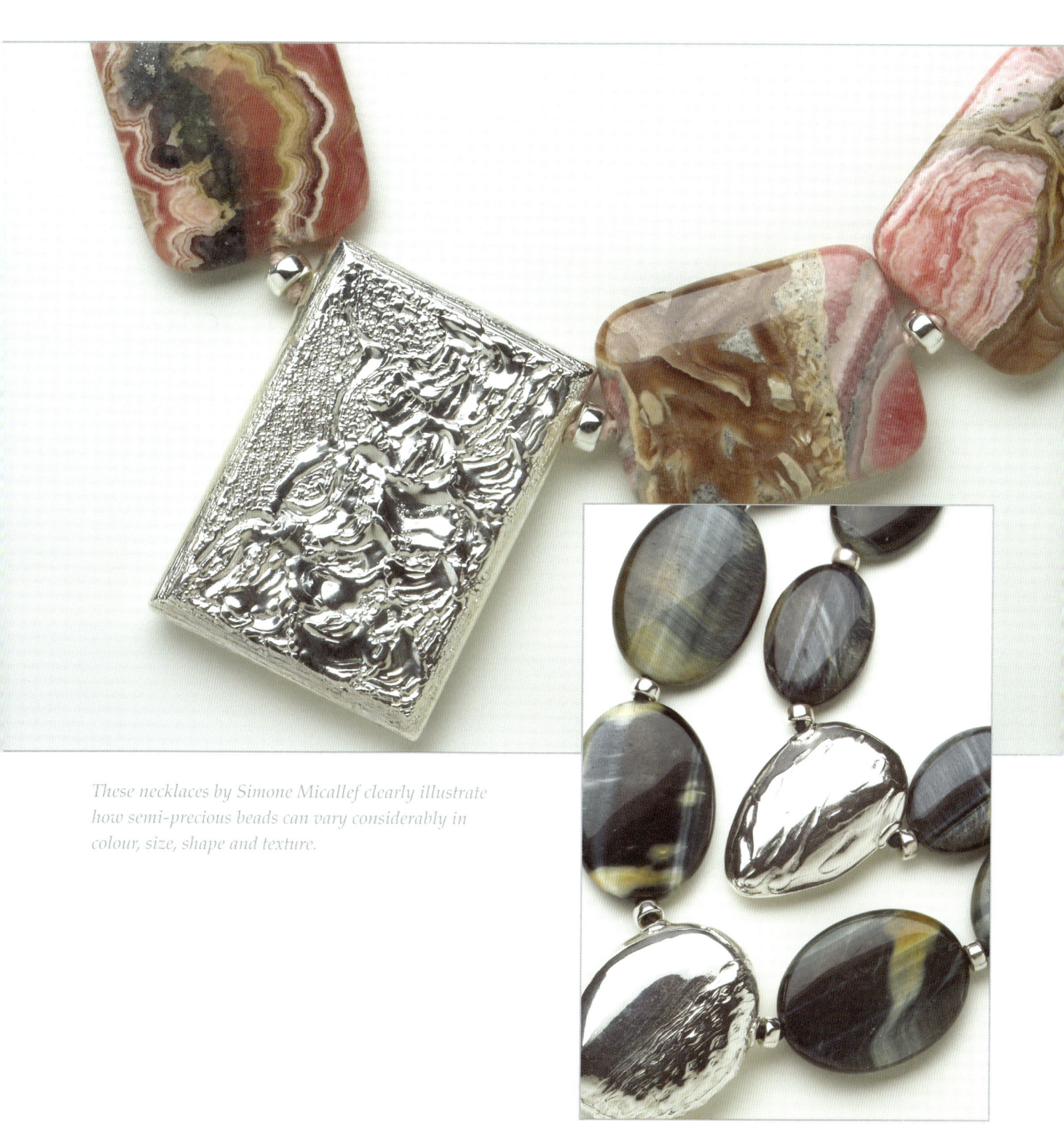

These necklaces by Simone Micallef clearly illustrate how semi-precious beads can vary considerably in colour, size, shape and texture.

53

Does This Look Good On Me?

Glass beads

Wearing jewellery made from glass beads is a fabulous way to inject colour into an outfit. Beads are often inexpensive and available in every High Street. Individually designed, handmade bead jewellery adds that something special, as it is not only the colour and combination of colour used that is different from the High Street, but that each bead is unique.

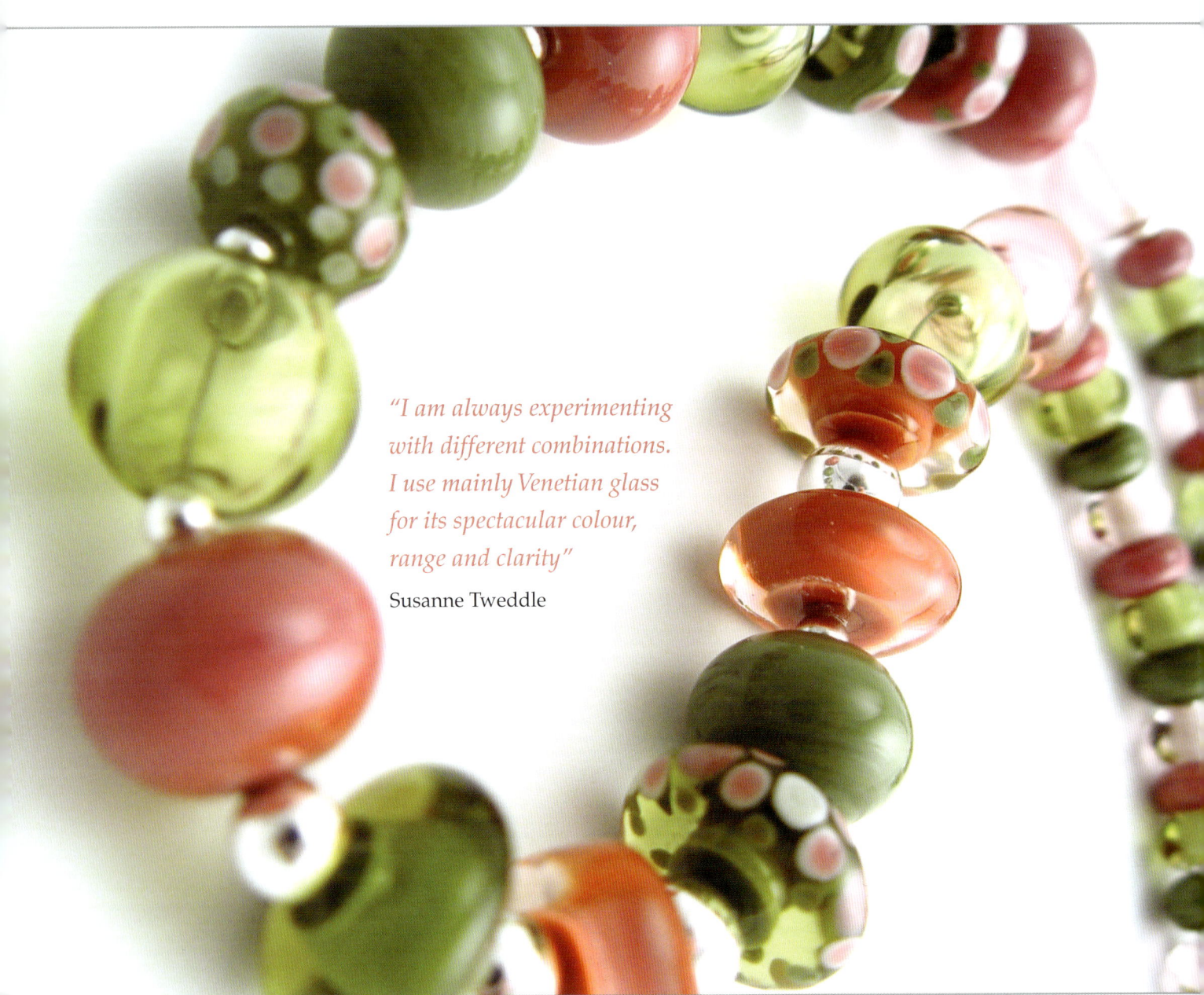

"I am always experimenting with different combinations. I use mainly Venetian glass for its spectacular colour, range and clarity"

Susanne Tweddle

Chapter Six: Colour

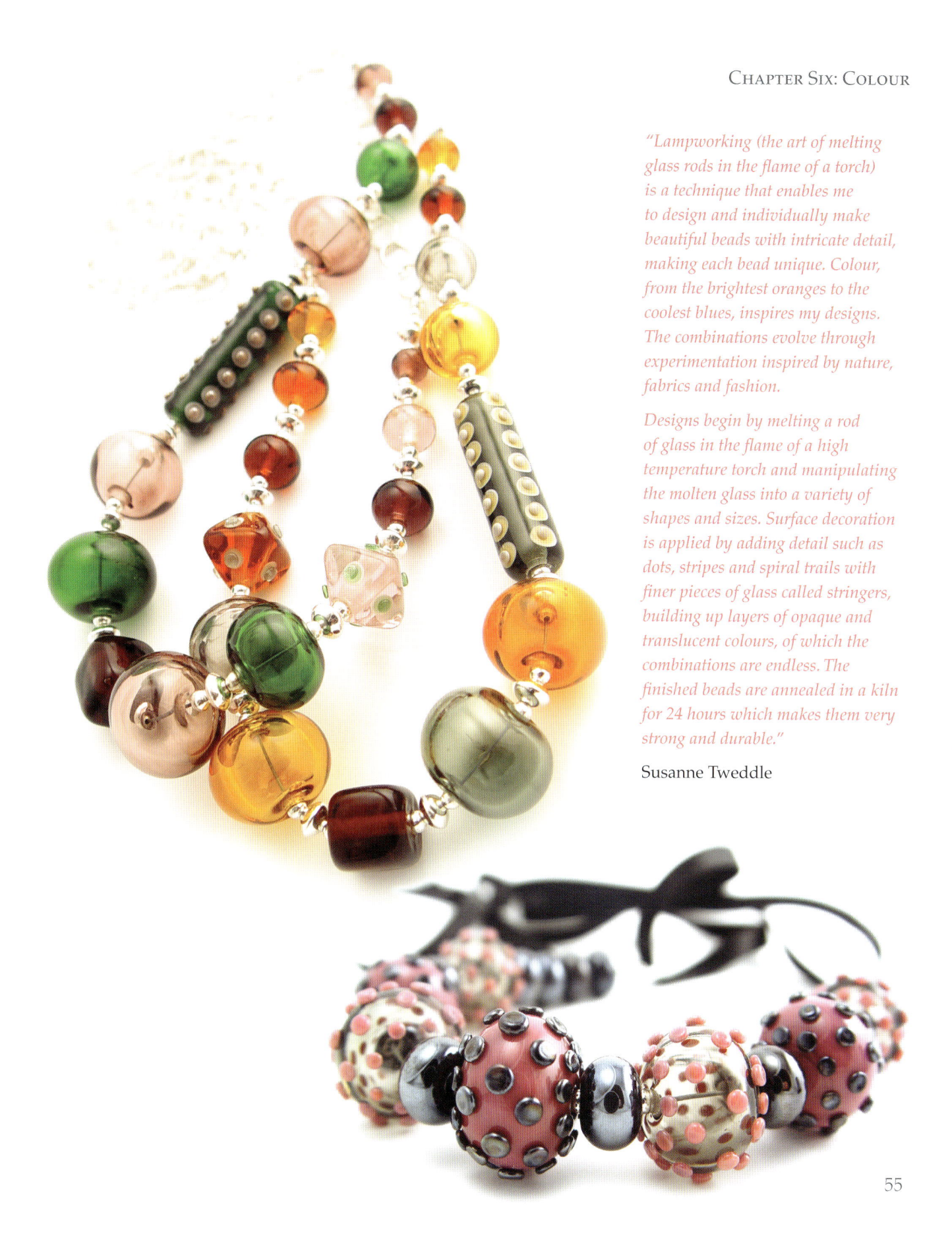

"Lampworking (the art of melting glass rods in the flame of a torch) is a technique that enables me to design and individually make beautiful beads with intricate detail, making each bead unique. Colour, from the brightest oranges to the coolest blues, inspires my designs. The combinations evolve through experimentation inspired by nature, fabrics and fashion.

Designs begin by melting a rod of glass in the flame of a high temperature torch and manipulating the molten glass into a variety of shapes and sizes. Surface decoration is applied by adding detail such as dots, stripes and spiral trails with finer pieces of glass called stringers, building up layers of opaque and translucent colours, of which the combinations are endless. The finished beads are annealed in a kiln for 24 hours which makes them very strong and durable."

Susanne Tweddle

DOES THIS LOOK GOOD ON ME?

Anodised Aluminuim

Aluminum is a silver coloured metal which is inexpensive when compared to silver. It does not rust, is malleable and is lightweight. Carole Allen uses aluminum to make brightly coloured jewellery. She describes the process in the account which follows:

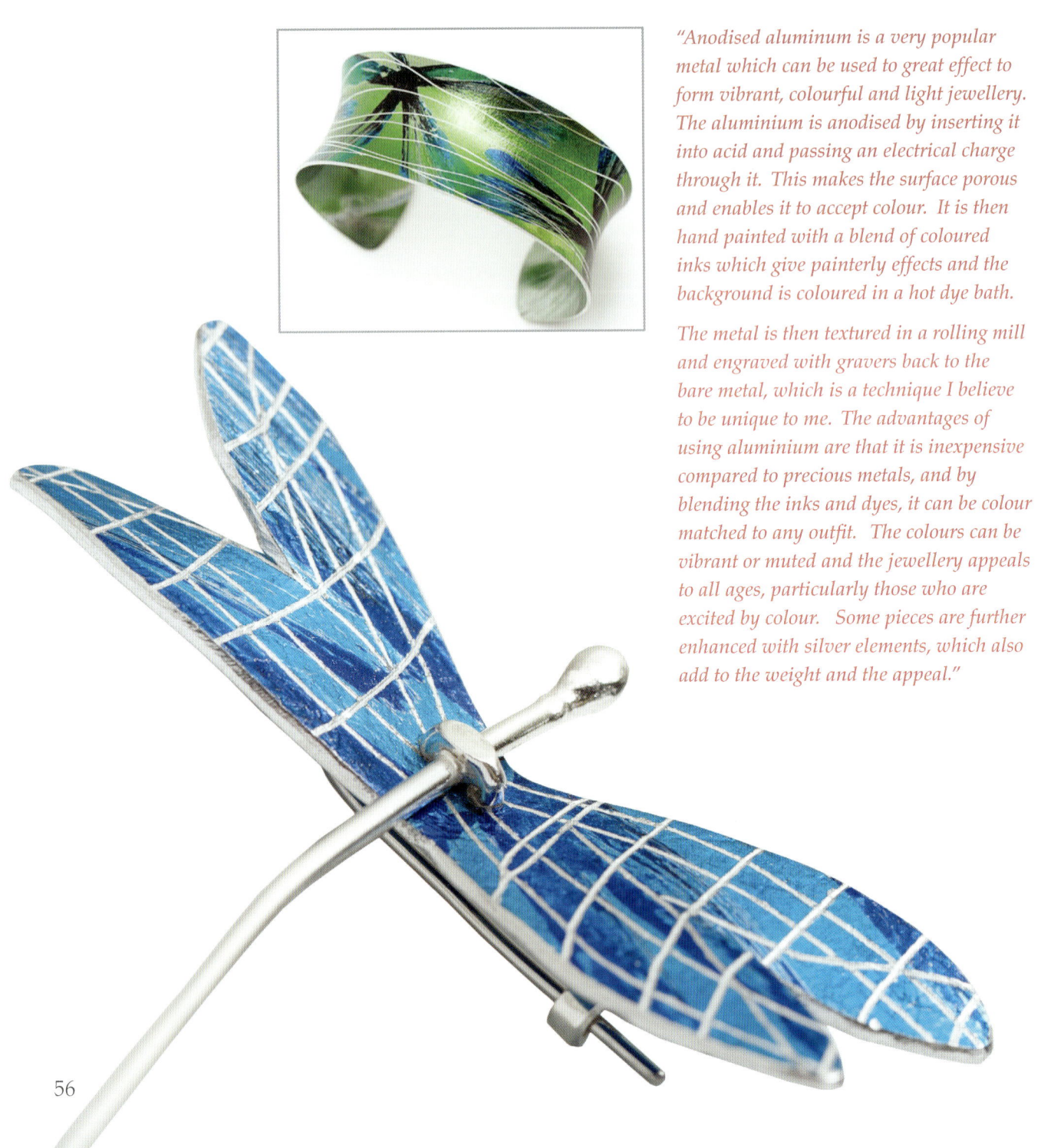

"Anodised aluminum is a very popular metal which can be used to great effect to form vibrant, colourful and light jewellery. The aluminium is anodised by inserting it into acid and passing an electrical charge through it. This makes the surface porous and enables it to accept colour. It is then hand painted with a blend of coloured inks which give painterly effects and the background is coloured in a hot dye bath.

The metal is then textured in a rolling mill and engraved with gravers back to the bare metal, which is a technique I believe to be unique to me. The advantages of using aluminium are that it is inexpensive compared to precious metals, and by blending the inks and dyes, it can be colour matched to any outfit. The colours can be vibrant or muted and the jewellery appeals to all ages, particularly those who are excited by colour. Some pieces are further enhanced with silver elements, which also add to the weight and the appeal."

CHAPTER SIX: COLOUR

Plastics, perspex and acrylics are materials that are becoming more and more popular with the designer maker. Acrylic jewellery has been added to Carole Allen's portfolio in her efforts to add colour to her work, whilst keeping her work affordable to her customers.

Coloured plastics & acrylics

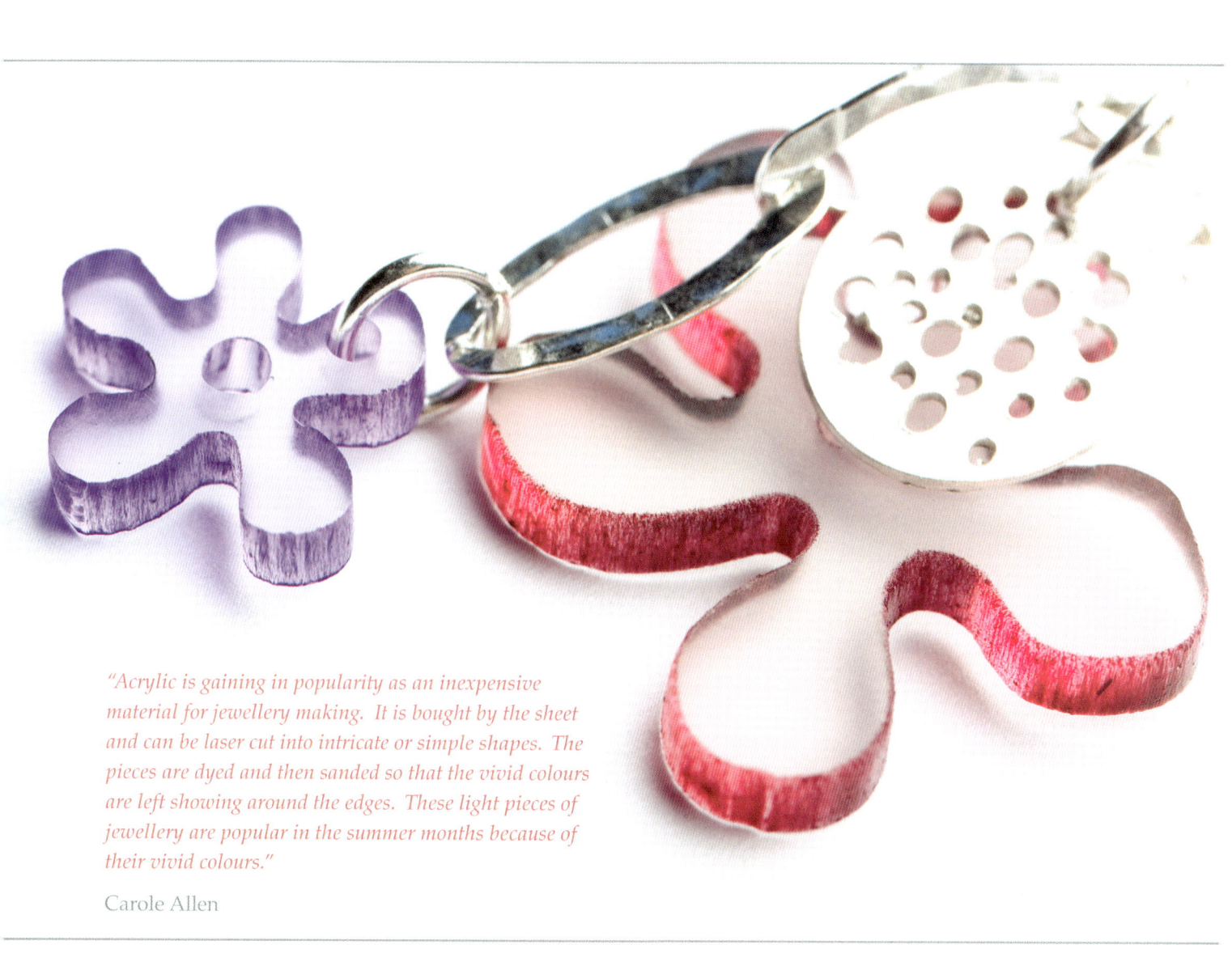

"Acrylic is gaining in popularity as an inexpensive material for jewellery making. It is bought by the sheet and can be laser cut into intricate or simple shapes. The pieces are dyed and then sanded so that the vivid colours are left showing around the edges. These light pieces of jewellery are popular in the summer months because of their vivid colours."

Carole Allen

57

Does This Look Good On Me?

Coloured textiles

Textiles are being used much more to produce exciting and vibrant jewellery. Felts, laces and silks have all be used extensively, but it is possible to make jewellery from any type of fabric.

Liz Willis combines the idea of using textiles to make jewellery with the more conventional metal techniques to produce contemporary jewellery with a difference.

Liz uses silver and gold wire to form appropriate shapes and then hand stitches over part or all of it with silk threads, occasionally using pearls or semi-precious stones or glass beads, to add to the colour and texture.

Chapter Six: Colour

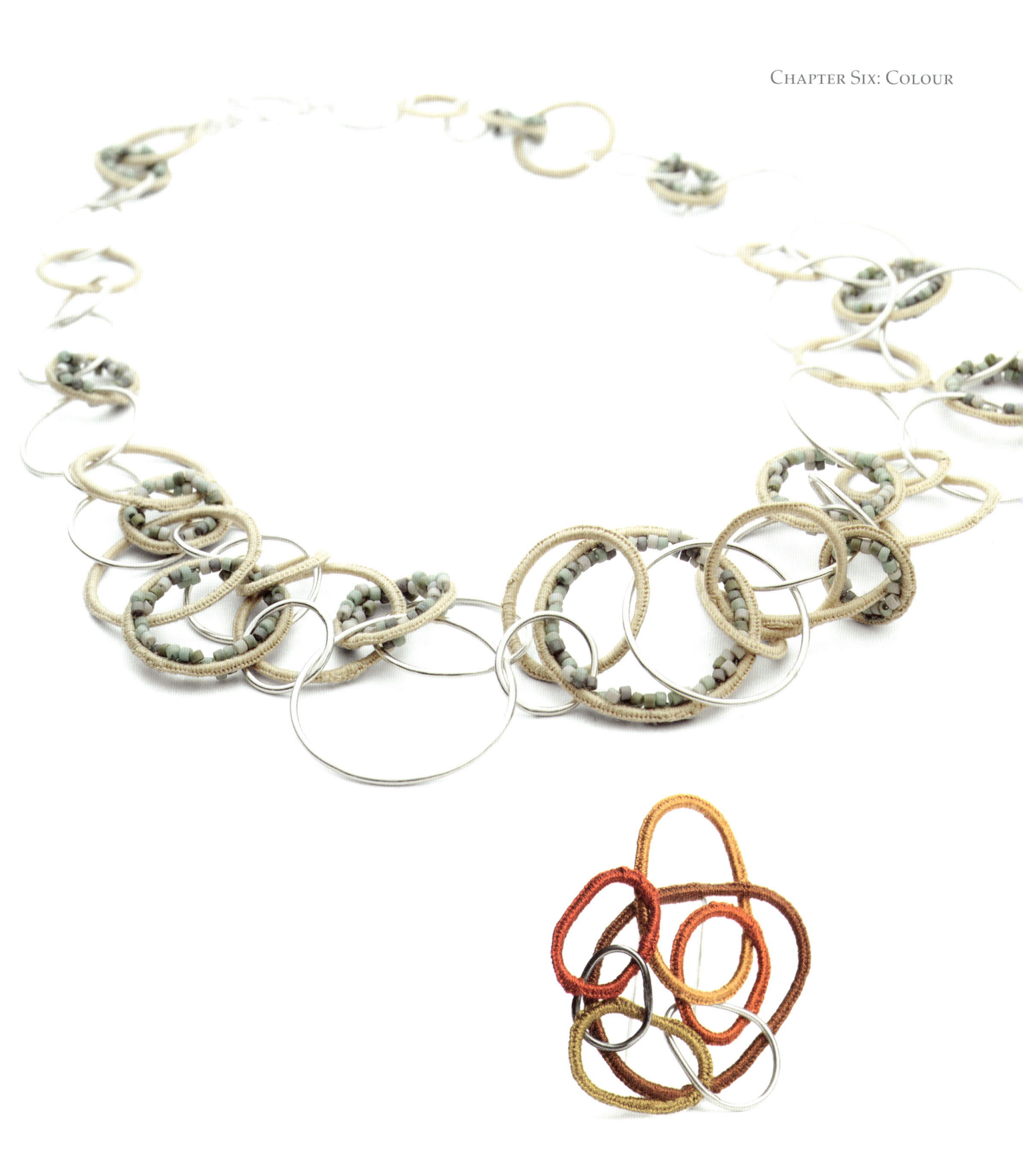

DOES THIS LOOK GOOD ON ME?

Mixed metal jewellery

Jewellery can be made more colourful by making it with metals of different colours, or by treating the surface of the metal with heat or chemicals.

"Adding gold to silver jewellery is becoming increasingly popular. Much of my jewellery is a mixture of silver and gold. My reasons for including the two metals are to produce a contrast in colour and more importantly to enable my jewellery to look good on everyone. The jewellery I make is predominantly silver so tends to suit those who look good in silver. To enable those who suit gold to wear my work I have added gold to some jewellery ranges. My popular Classic Leaf range is a good example of a jewellery range which looks good on most people, as it is available in silver only or with varying amounts of gold."

Karen Faulkner-Dunkley

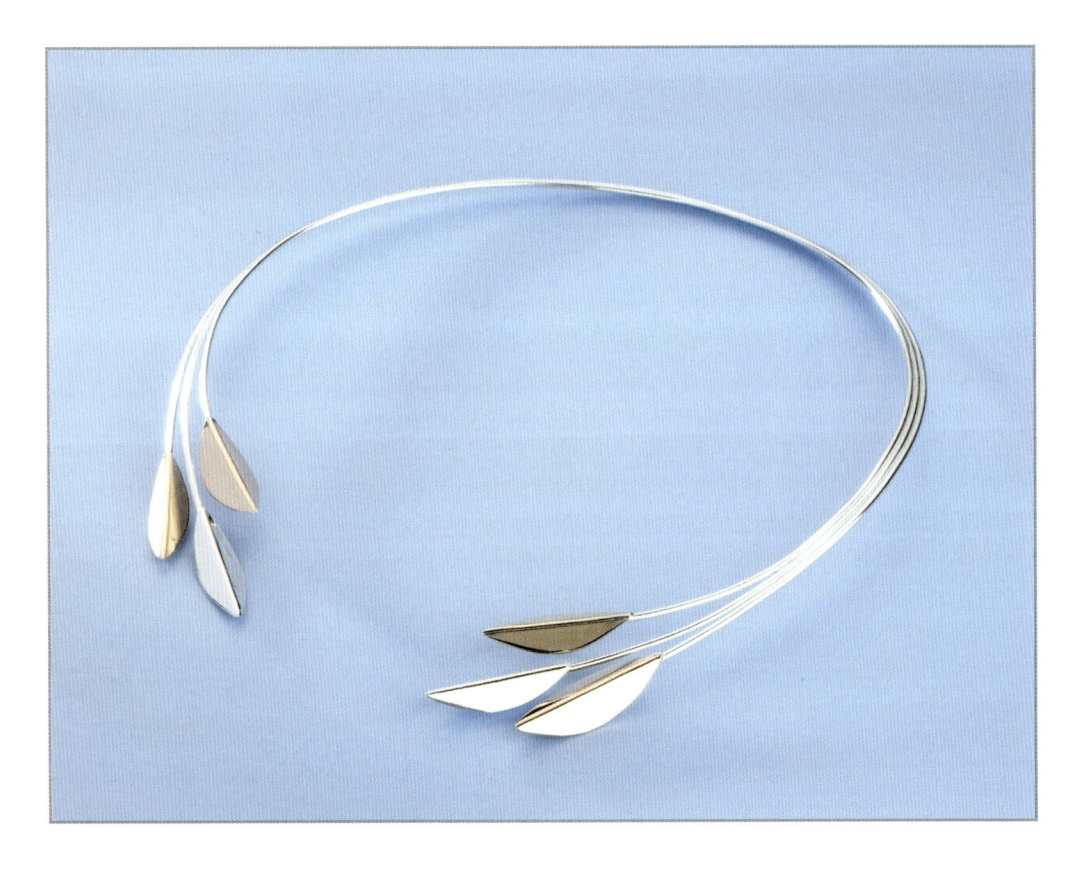

KFD Jewellery Classic Leaf Torque in silver and 9ct rose and yellow golds

CHAPTER SIX: COLOUR

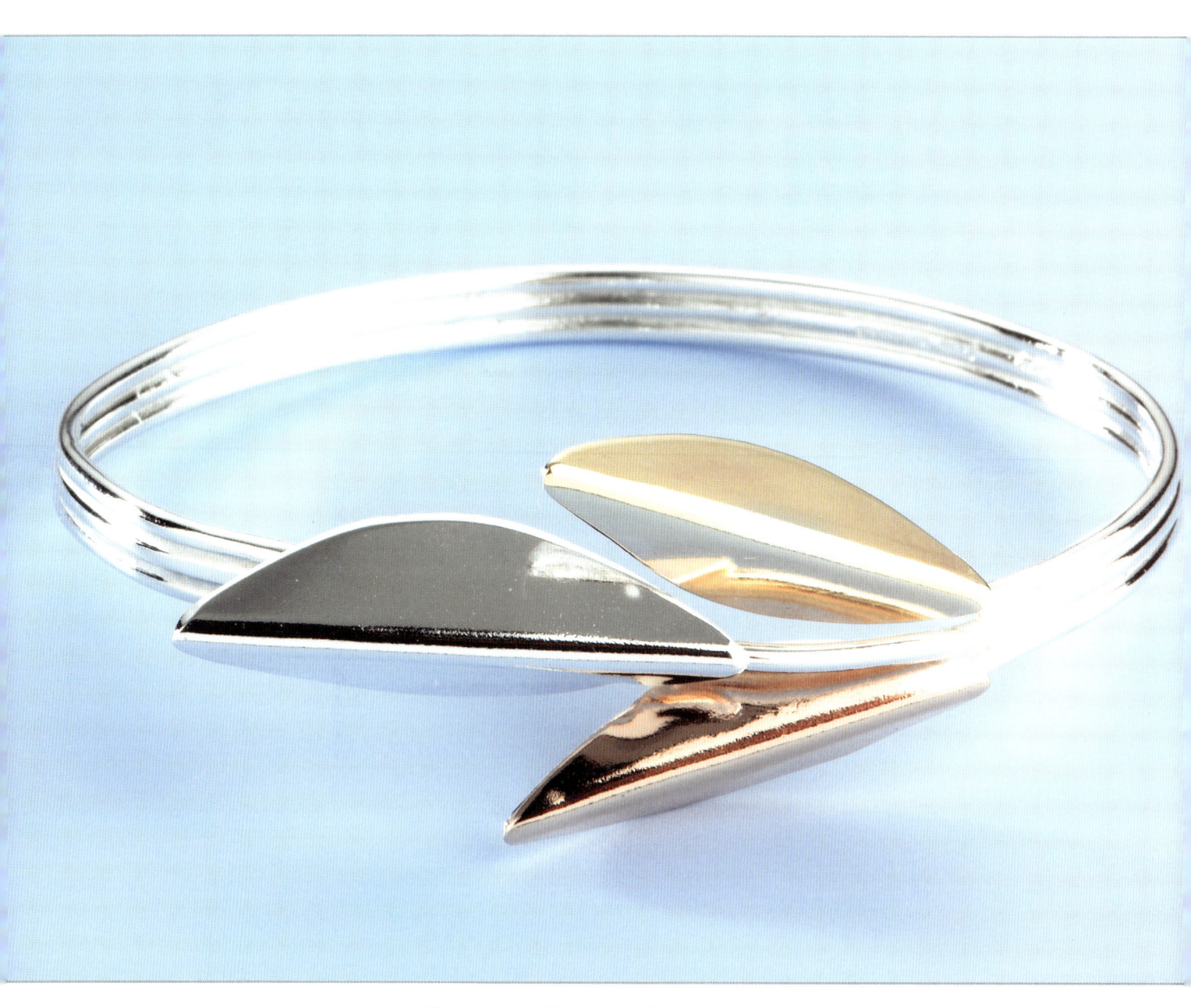

KFD Jewellery Classic Leaf Bangle in silver and 9ct rose and yellow golds

Does This Look Good On Me?

Changing the surface colour of metal

Metals can be treated with heat or chemicals, or they can be plated to change the colour and finish of the metal. The three rings in Hannah Souter's etched range (below) clearly illustrate how essentially the same ring can look very different by varying the surface finish of the metal. The matt silver effect has been produced by repeatedly heating and pickling the silver in dilute sulphuric acid or safety pickle. The 22ct gold has been plated onto the silver using electroplating techniques. The grey colour seen on the largest ring is formed by using a chemical called liver of sulphur to oxidize the silver.

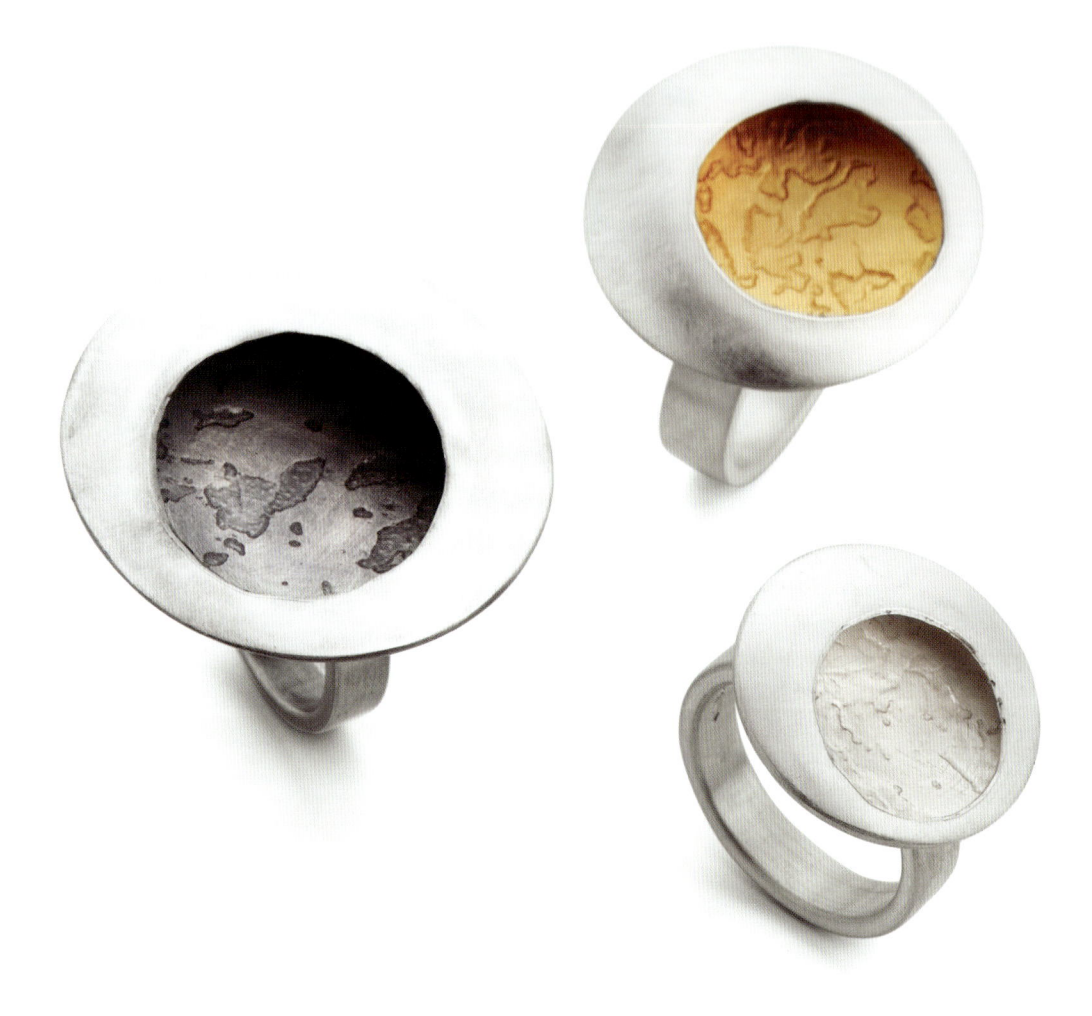

CHAPTER SIX: COLOUR

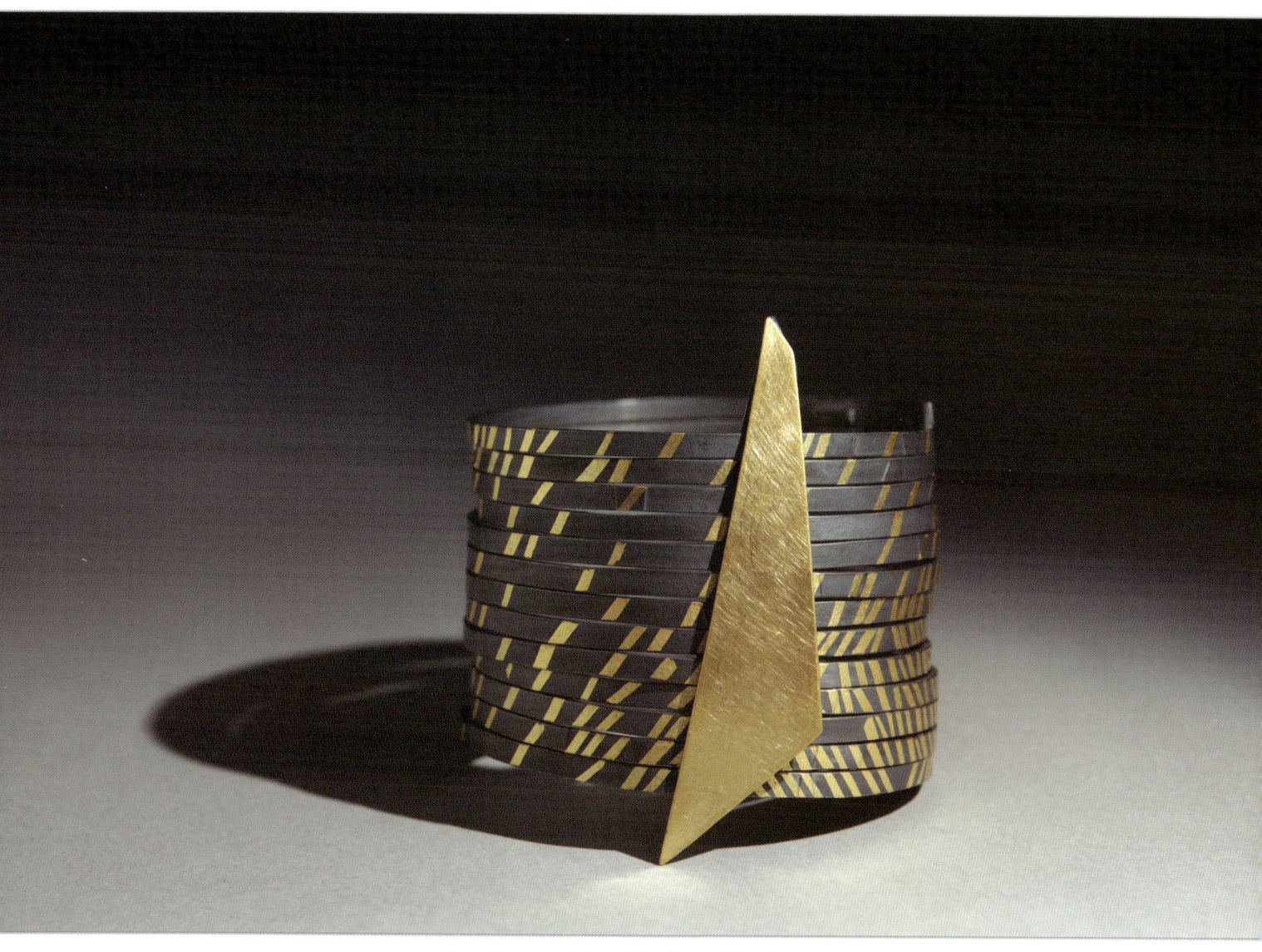

The silver in Shivani Patel's cuff has been completely oxidised to form a deep charcoal color, rather than the normal bright silver to produce a stronger, more dramatic contrast with the 24ct gold.

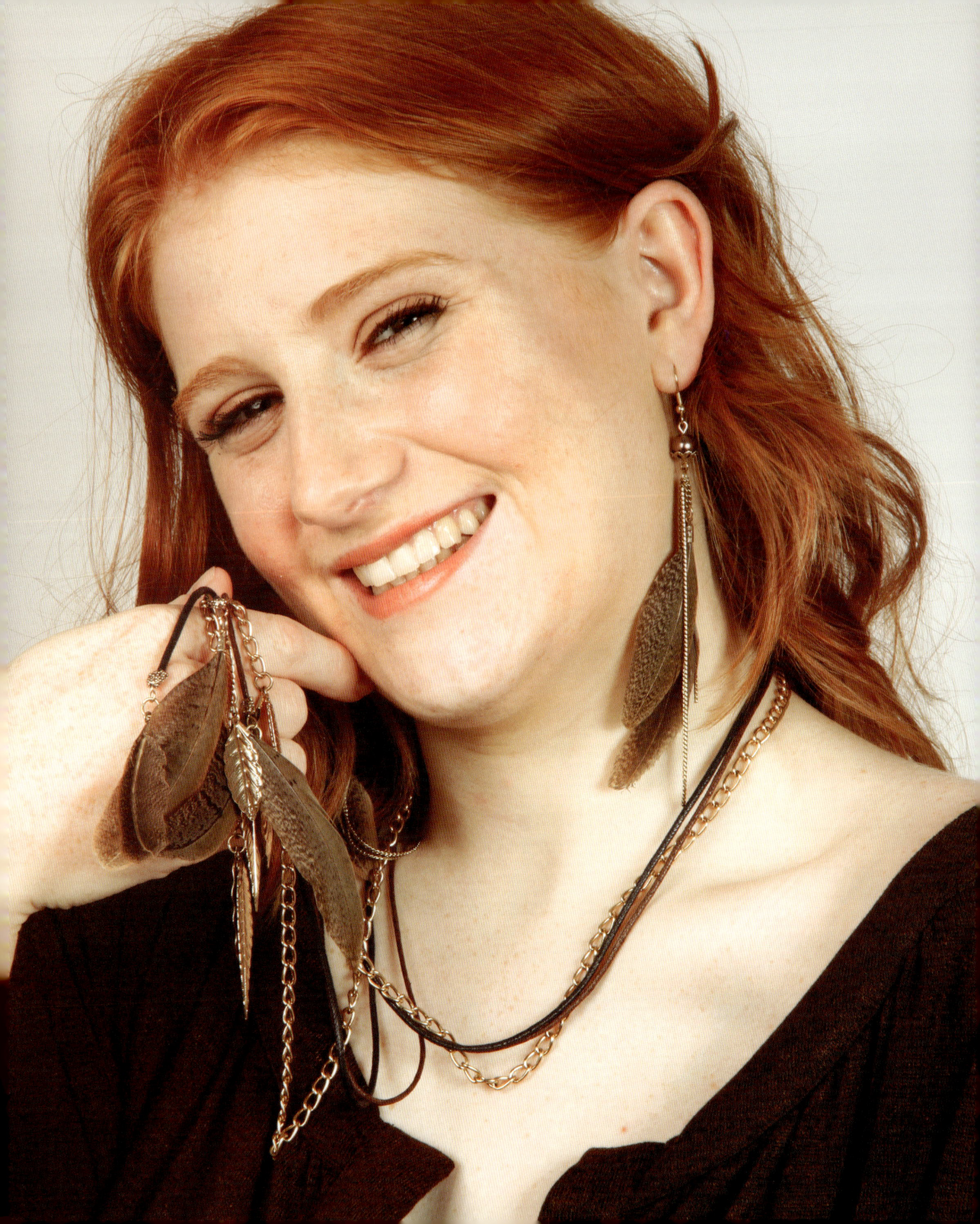

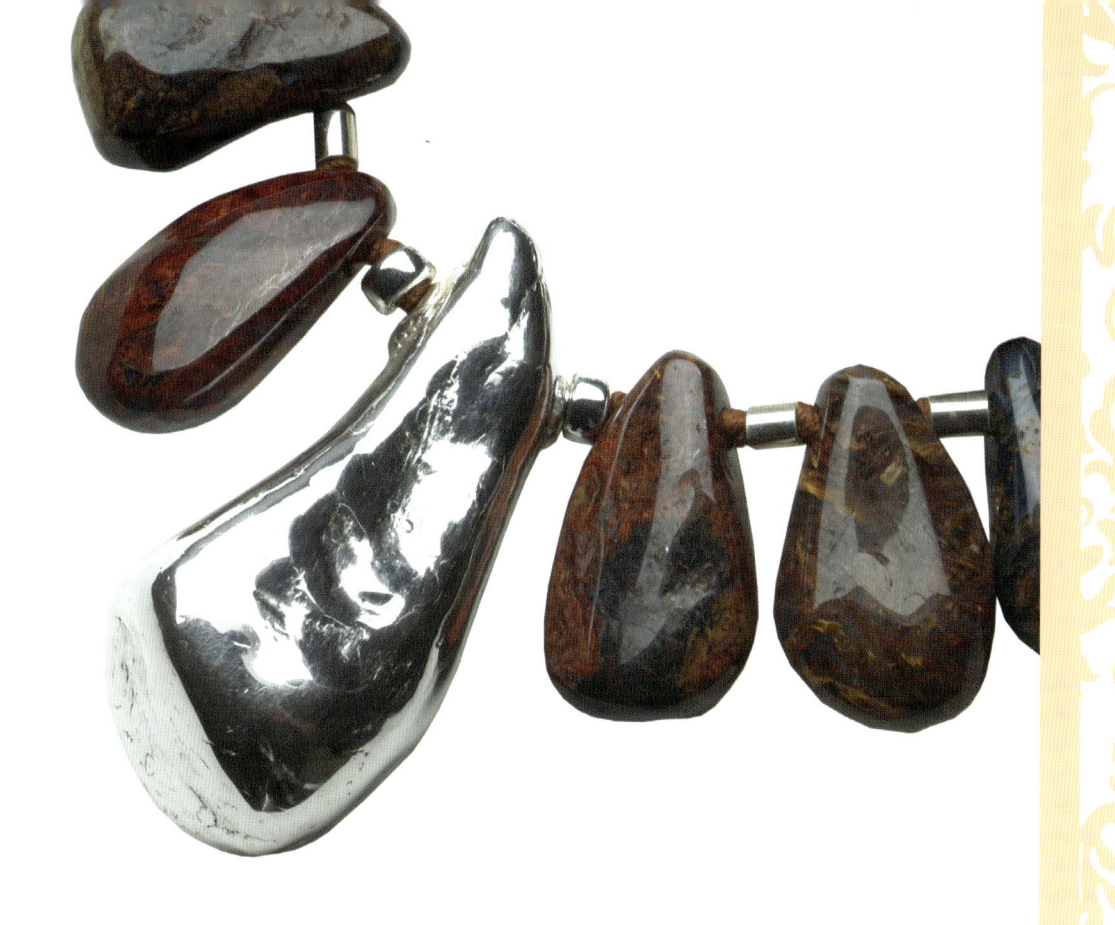

Chapter Seven

Personality

Does This Look Good On Me?

Personality

So far we have used our physical features to determine what jewellery looks best on us. We now need to take into account the fact that we are all unique individuals with our own preferences and perception of self. Jewellery is intensely personal and the jewellery you choose to wear reflects not only self image, but also how you want others to view you. It is the final, small detail that finishes a look. Jewellery can completely change the effect of an outfit – make it perfect or leave it lacking. Your choice of jewellery is an indication of your personality. Jewellery can signify confidence, accomplishment and wealth. It can suggest whether you take life seriously, or take a fun, witty, whimsical pathway. The values important to you in life may also be alluded to by the jewellery you do or don't wear.

Although we are all different, we can all be placed into one of four main categories. Our choices may overlap into the different categories, but one will always dominate.

The four categories are:

- Classic style
- Romantic
- Creative
- Casual

Each of the four categories can contain both traditional and mainstream jewellery as well as contemporary designer jewellery.

CHAPTER SEVEN: PERSONALITY

Classic style

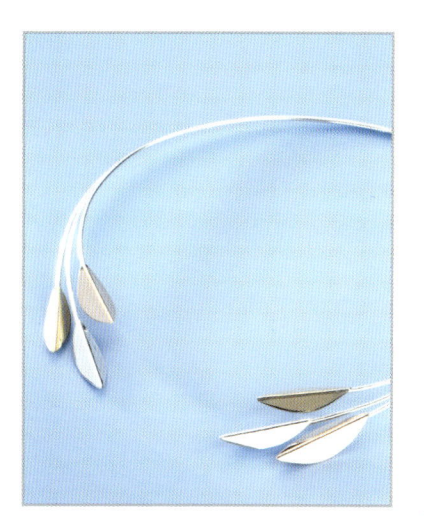

The Classic jewellery wearer is sophisticated and elegant. She likes stylish, uncluttered jewellery with clean lines and simple shapes. She never wears too much jewellery, limiting herself to a few key pieces. During the day she will normally wear stud earrings, a necklace, brooch earrings or bracelet, but never all of these. Her jewellery is understated and unobtrusive. For evening functions or special occasions she will keep to one statement piece of jewellery.

Designers in this category include Karen Faulkner-Dunkley (KFD Jewellery), Rachel Gogerly, Hannah Souter, Daniela Dobesova and Shivani Patel

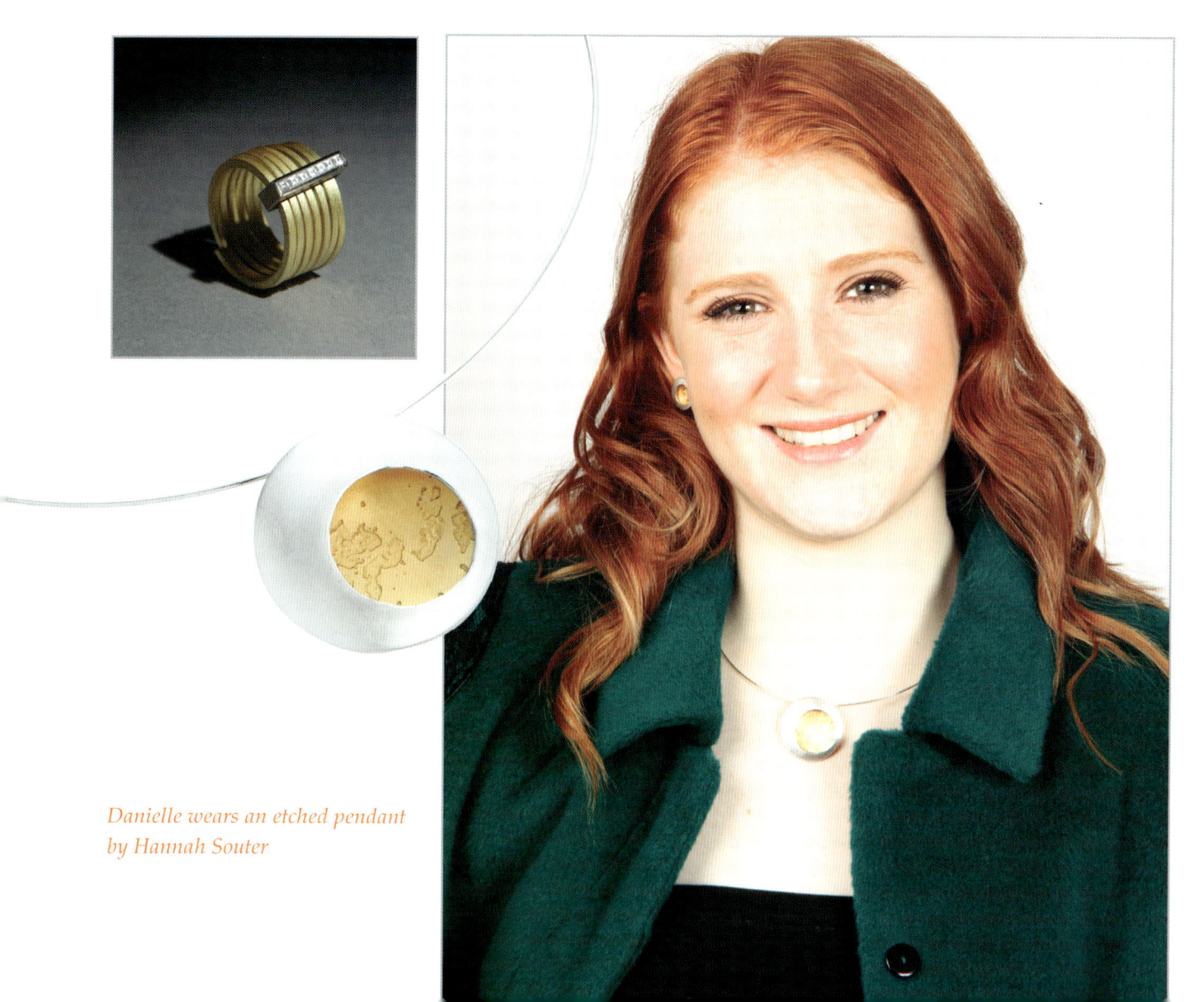

Danielle wears an etched pendant by Hannah Souter

Does This Look Good On Me?

Romantic

The Romantic jewellery wearer is very feminine. Her jewellery may be simple or fussy, but is always pretty. The jewellery often incorporates flowers, hearts and may signify a sentimental or deep meaning or tell a story. She may wear drop or stud earrings. Her bracelet may carry charms or have a message inscribed around it.

A selection of designers in this category include Lyn Antley, Susan Vedadi, Karen Faulkner-Dunkley (KFD Jewellery).

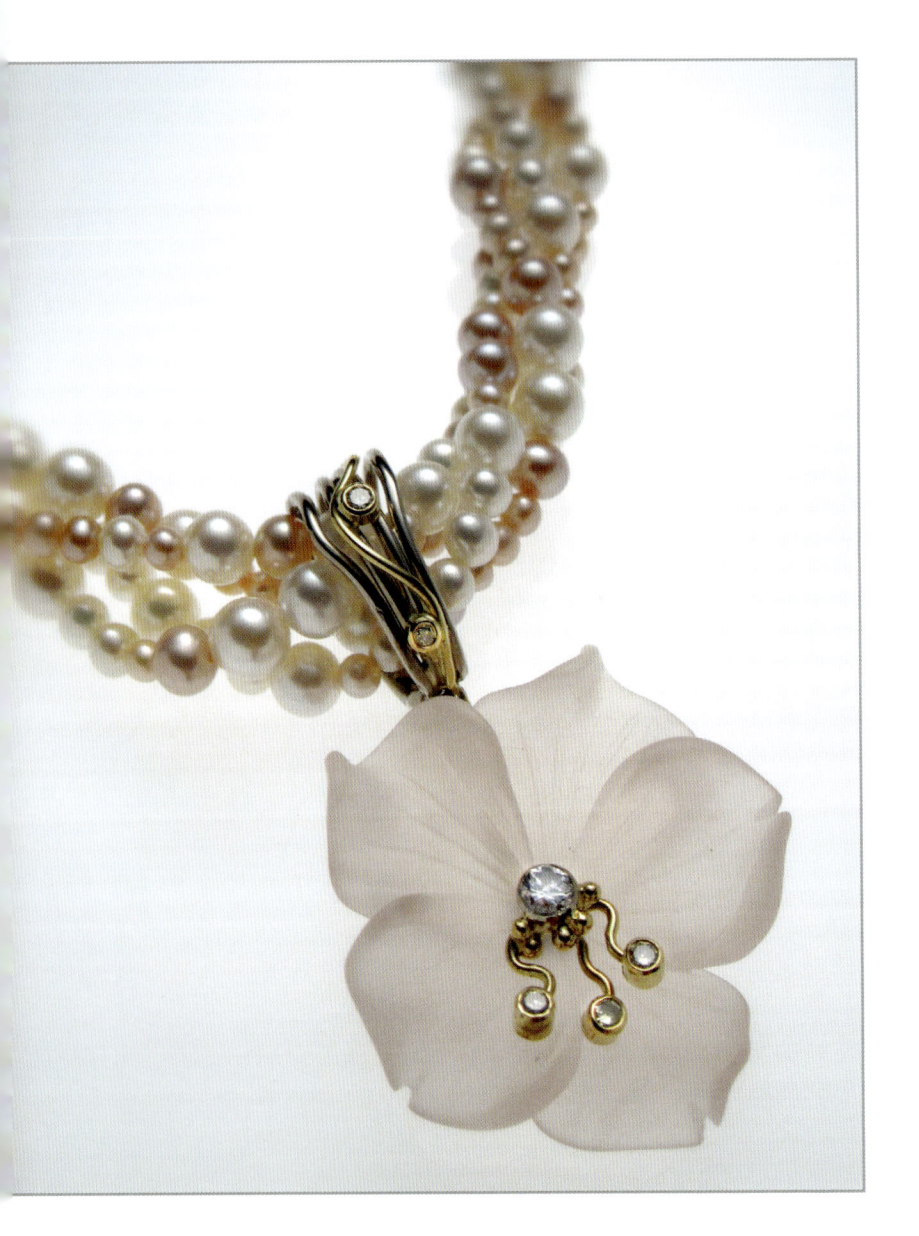

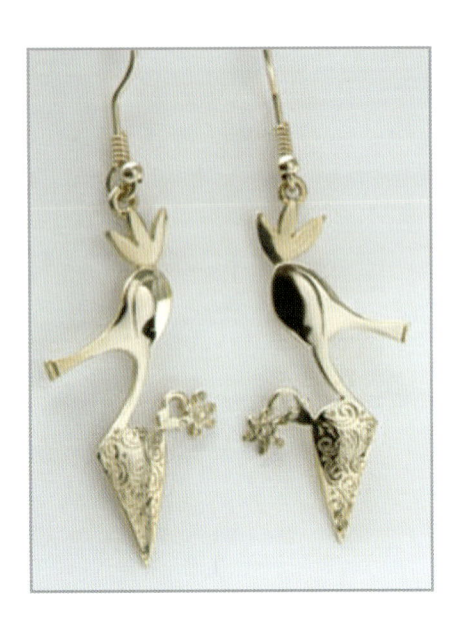

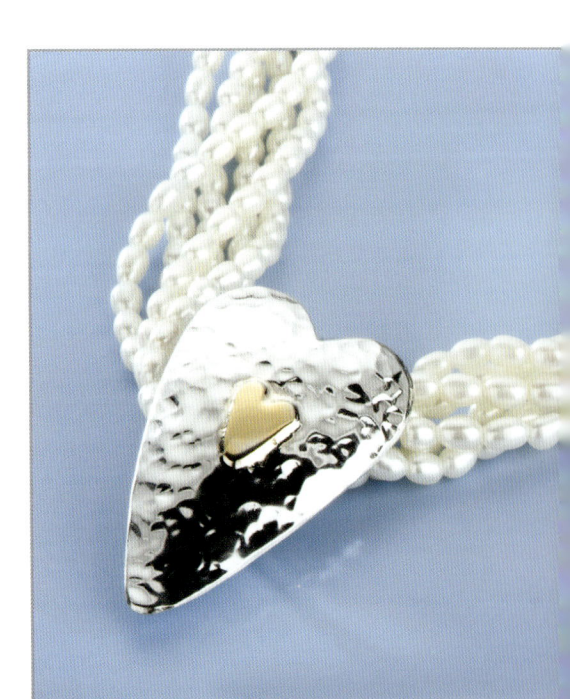

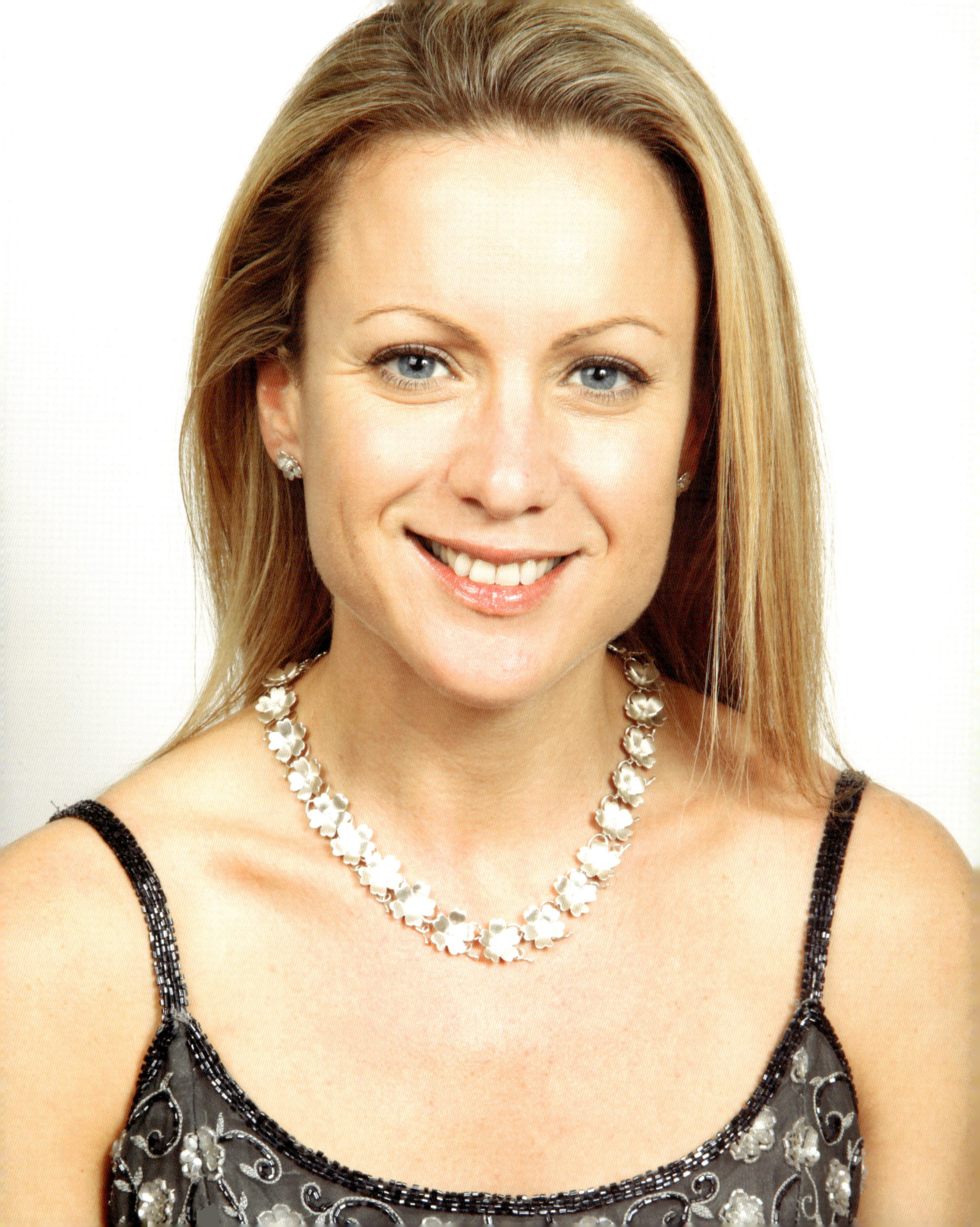

DOES THIS LOOK GOOD ON ME?

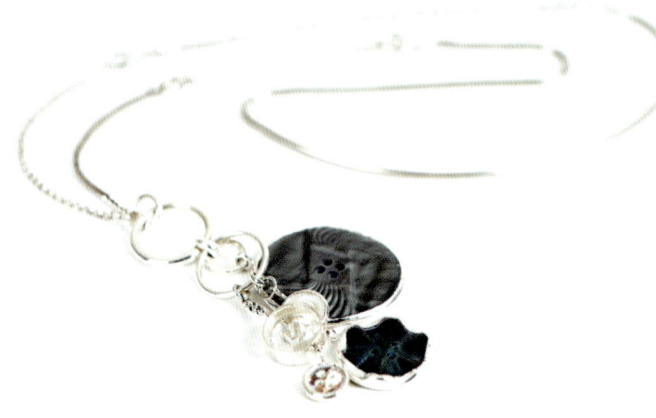

Creative The Creative jewellery wearer is very contemporary. She likes unique and different things. Her jewellery collection may be made from unconventional materials and may be very colourful. It often includes many statement jewellery pieces. She wants to be noticed and wants her jewellery to be noticed. This jewellery wearer may not wear much jewellery at the same time but what she does wear will be a statement.

Suggested creative designers are Lyn Antley, Shivani Patel, Emma Turpin, Carole Allen, Liz Willis, Karen Faulkner-Dunkley (KFD jewellery)

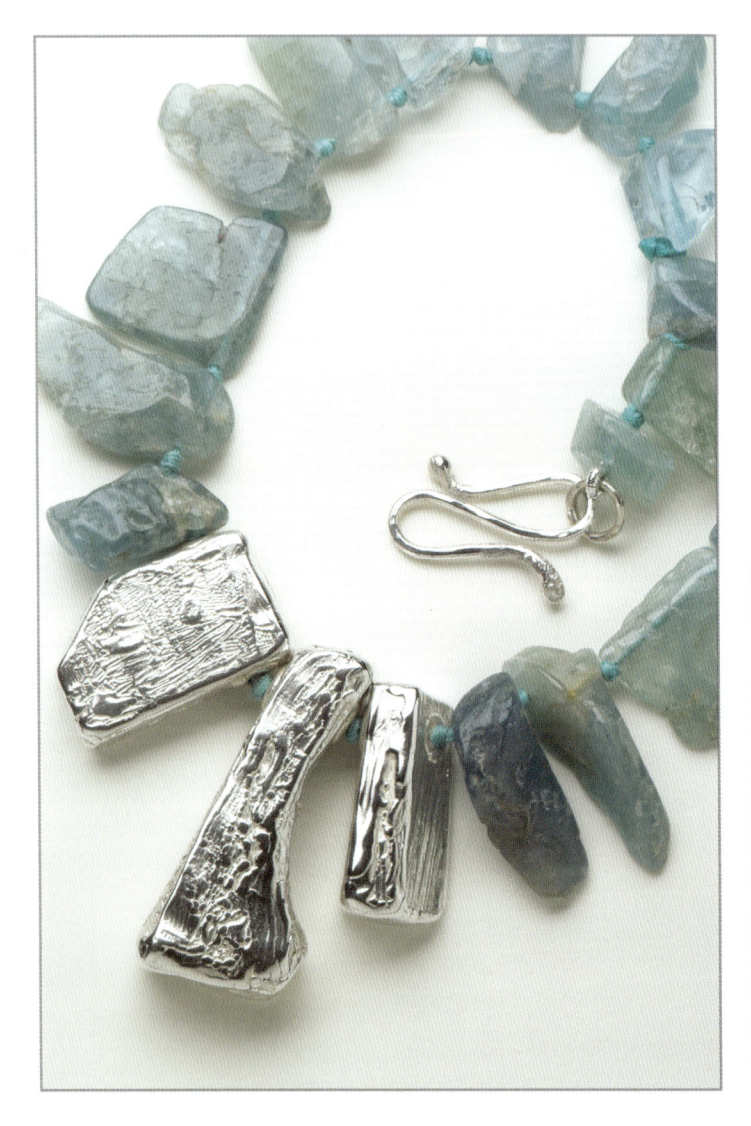

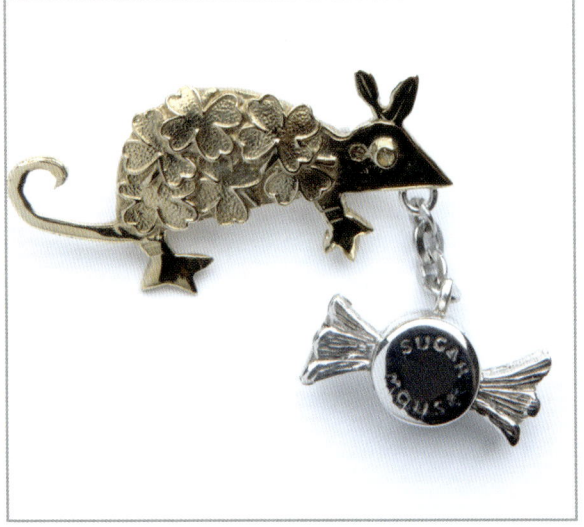

Chapter Seven: Personality

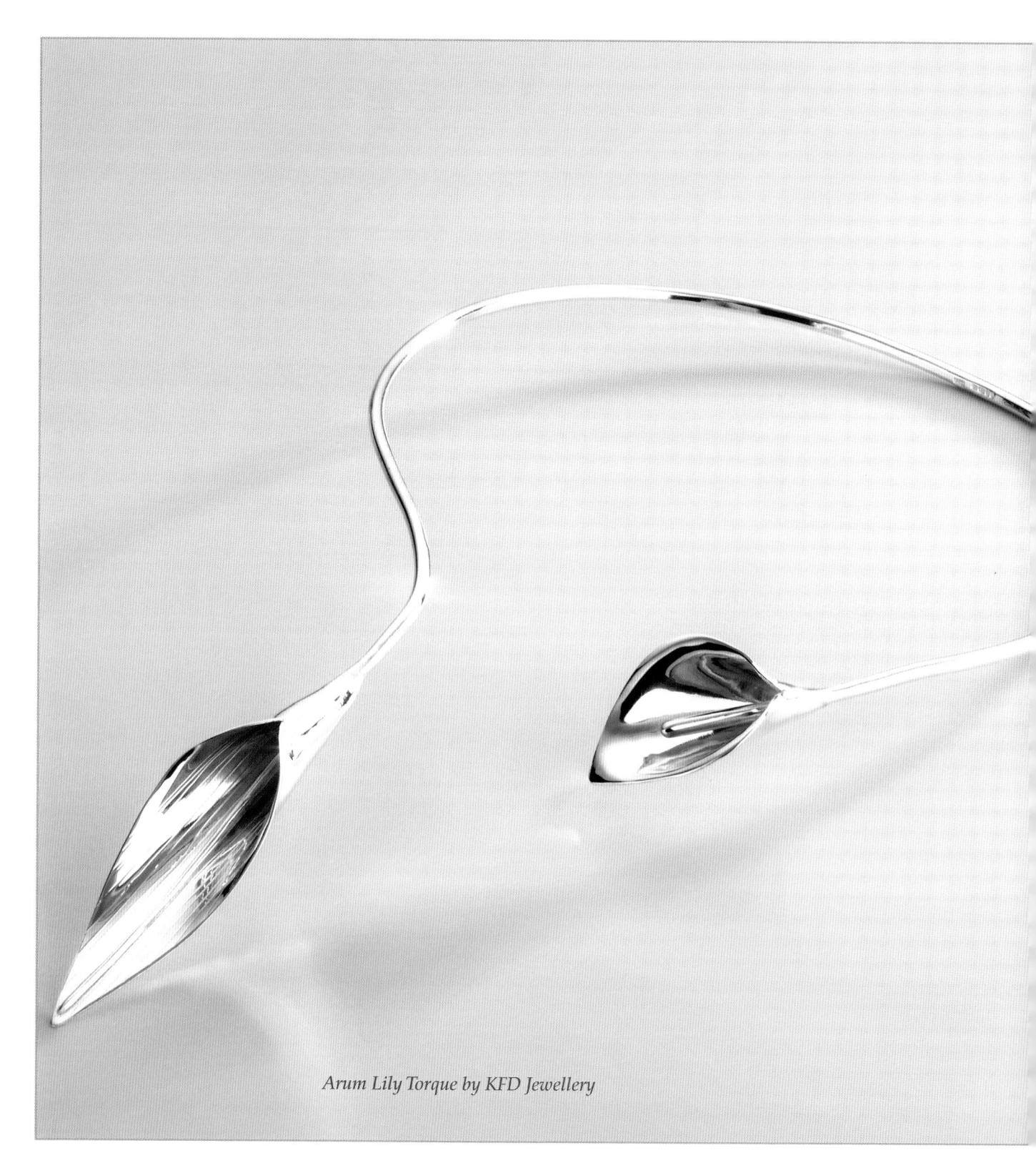

Arum Lily Torque by KFD Jewellery

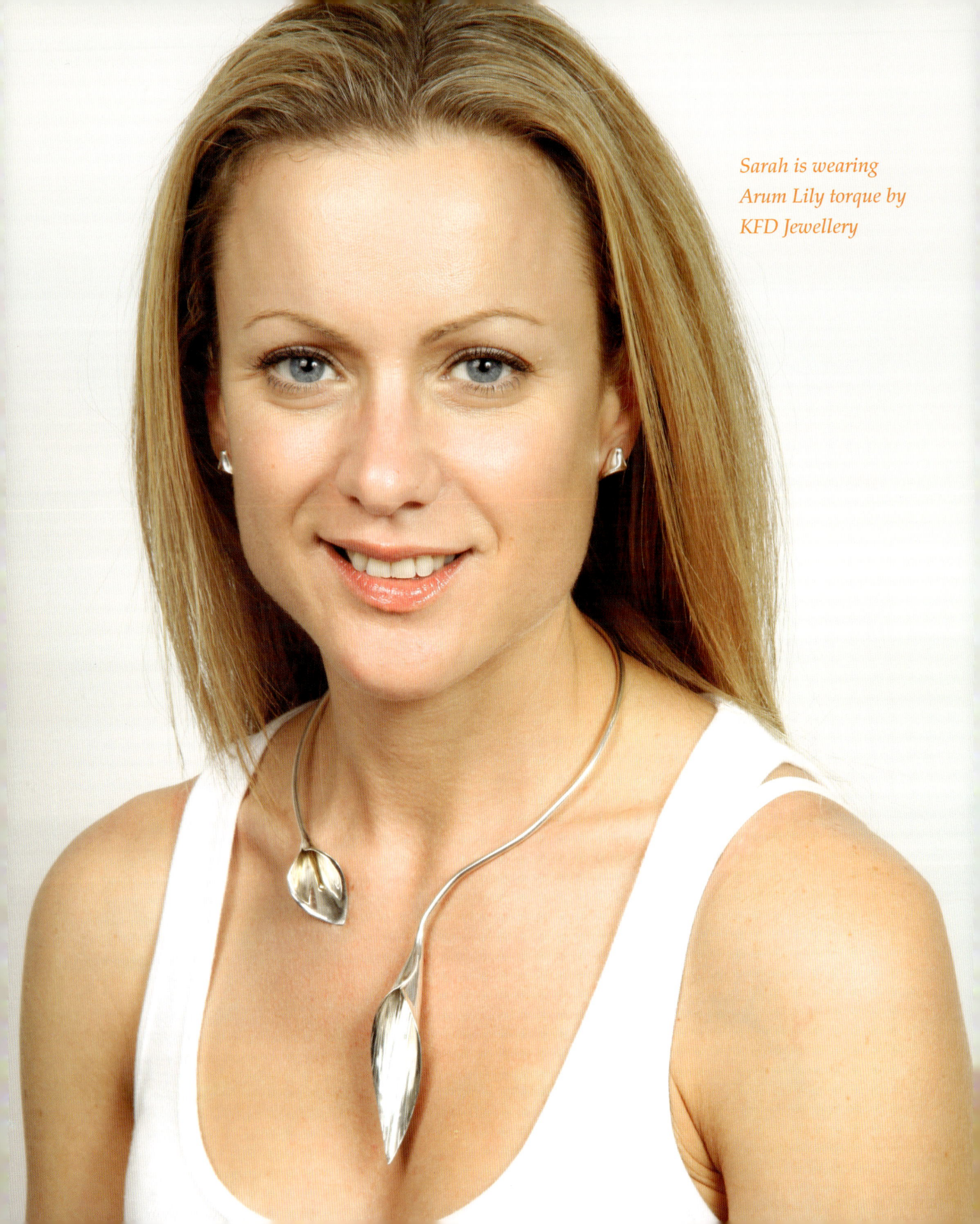

Sarah is wearing Arum Lily torque by KFD Jewellery

CHAPTER SEVEN: PERSONALITY

More examples of creative jewellery

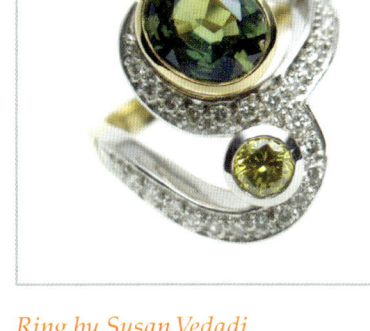

Ring by Susan Vedadi green sapphire, yellow and white diamonds

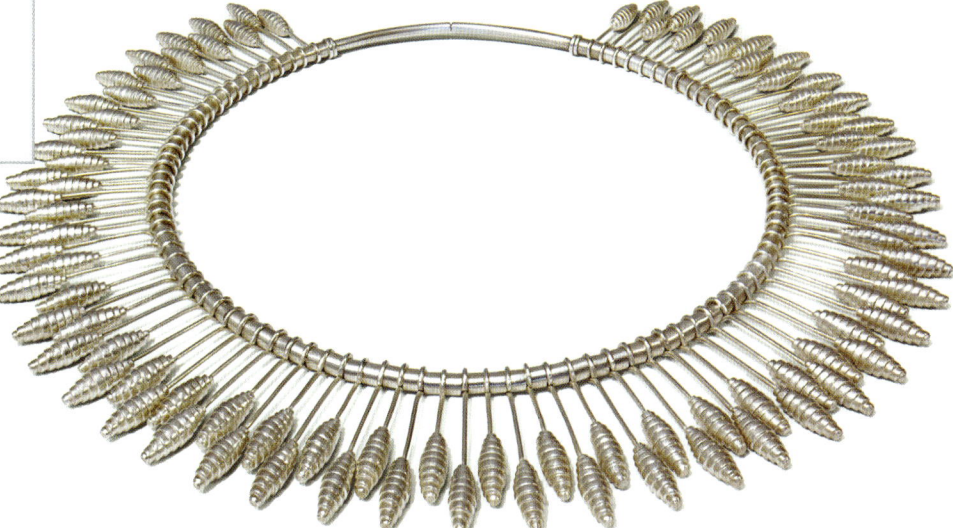

Ceres necklace by Daniela Dobesova

Anodised ring by Carole Allen

Frame ring by Emma Turpin

Casual   The Casual jewellery wearer is often very practical in nature and needs pieces which are easy to wear and which go with a lot of outfits. A few key pieces are all that are usually worn at any one time. This individual usually does not choose glitzy jewellery but prefers a relaxed feel, choosing simple metal, semiprecious beads or possibly wood instead.

Examples of casual designers are Simone Micallef, Heather Stowell, Liz Willis and Theresa Galanides

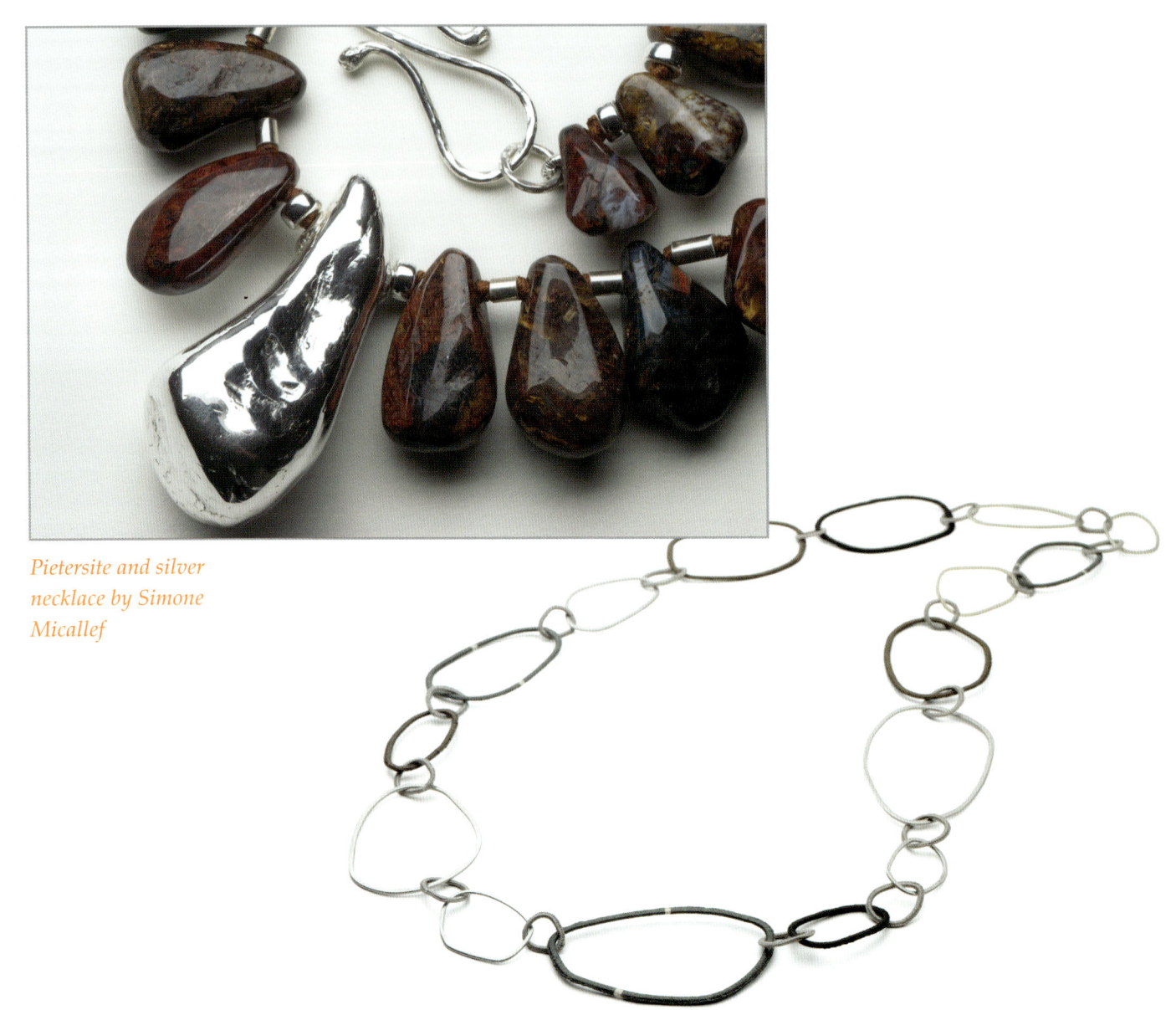

Pietersite and silver necklace by Simone Micallef

CHAPTER SEVEN: PERSONALITY

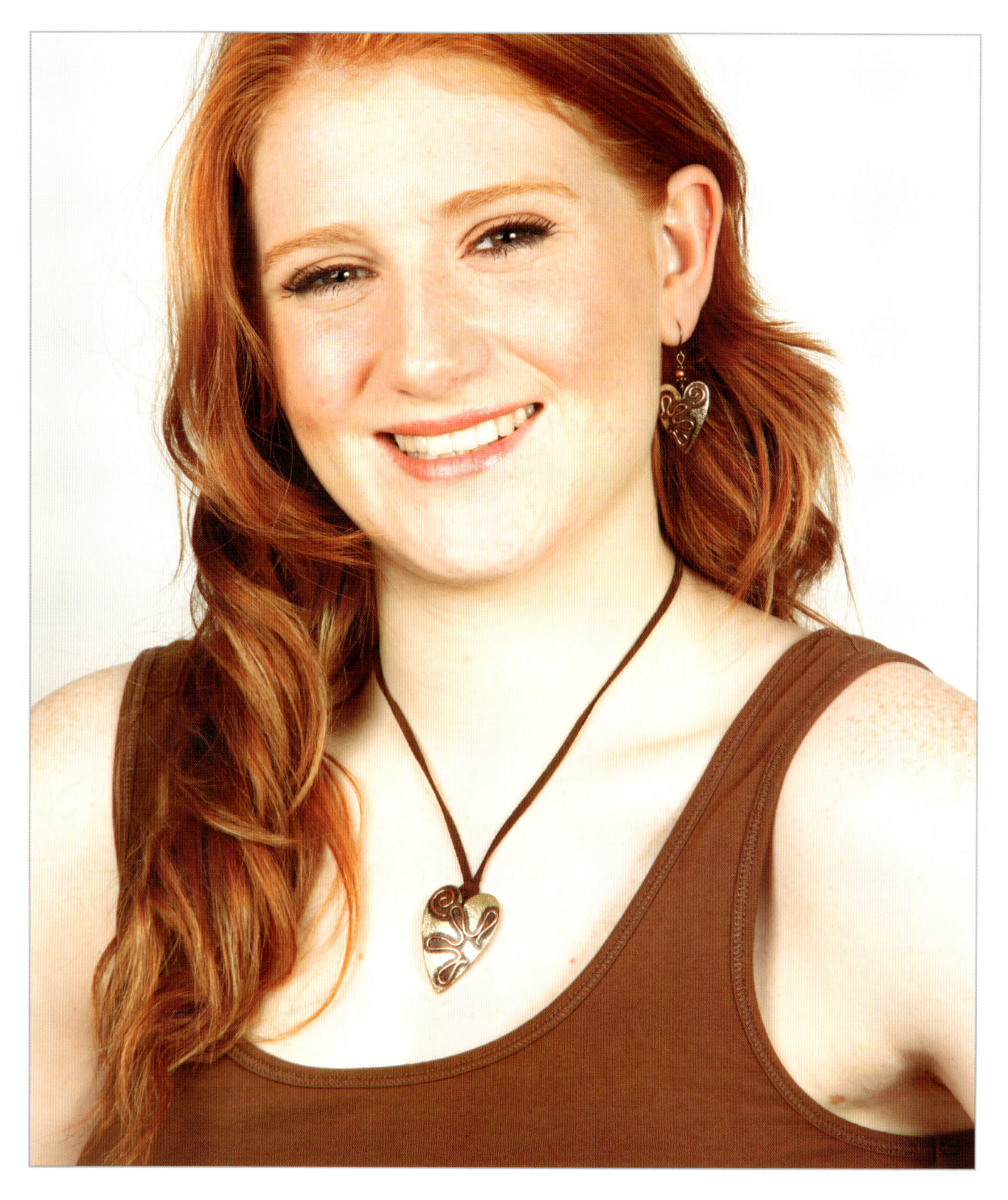

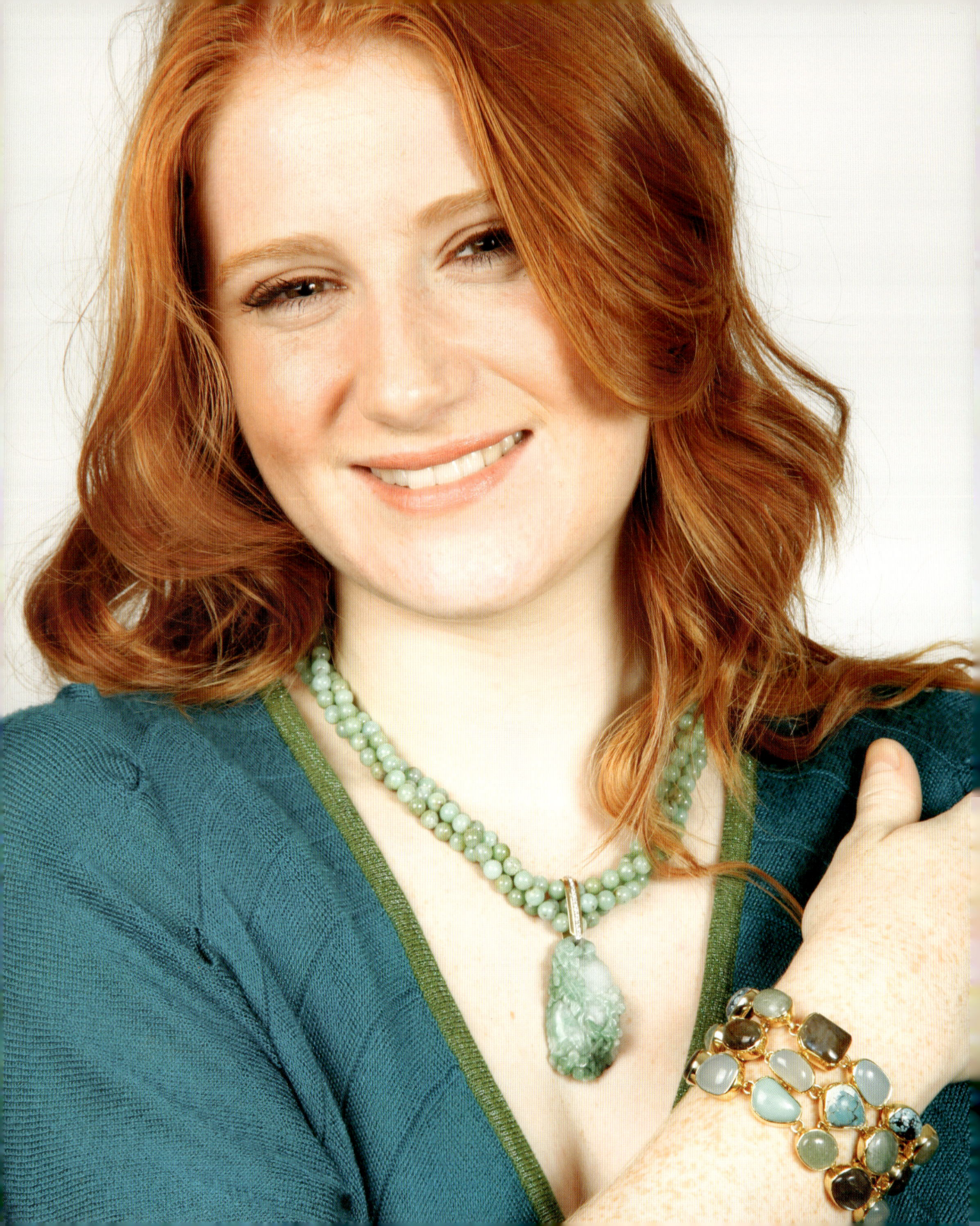

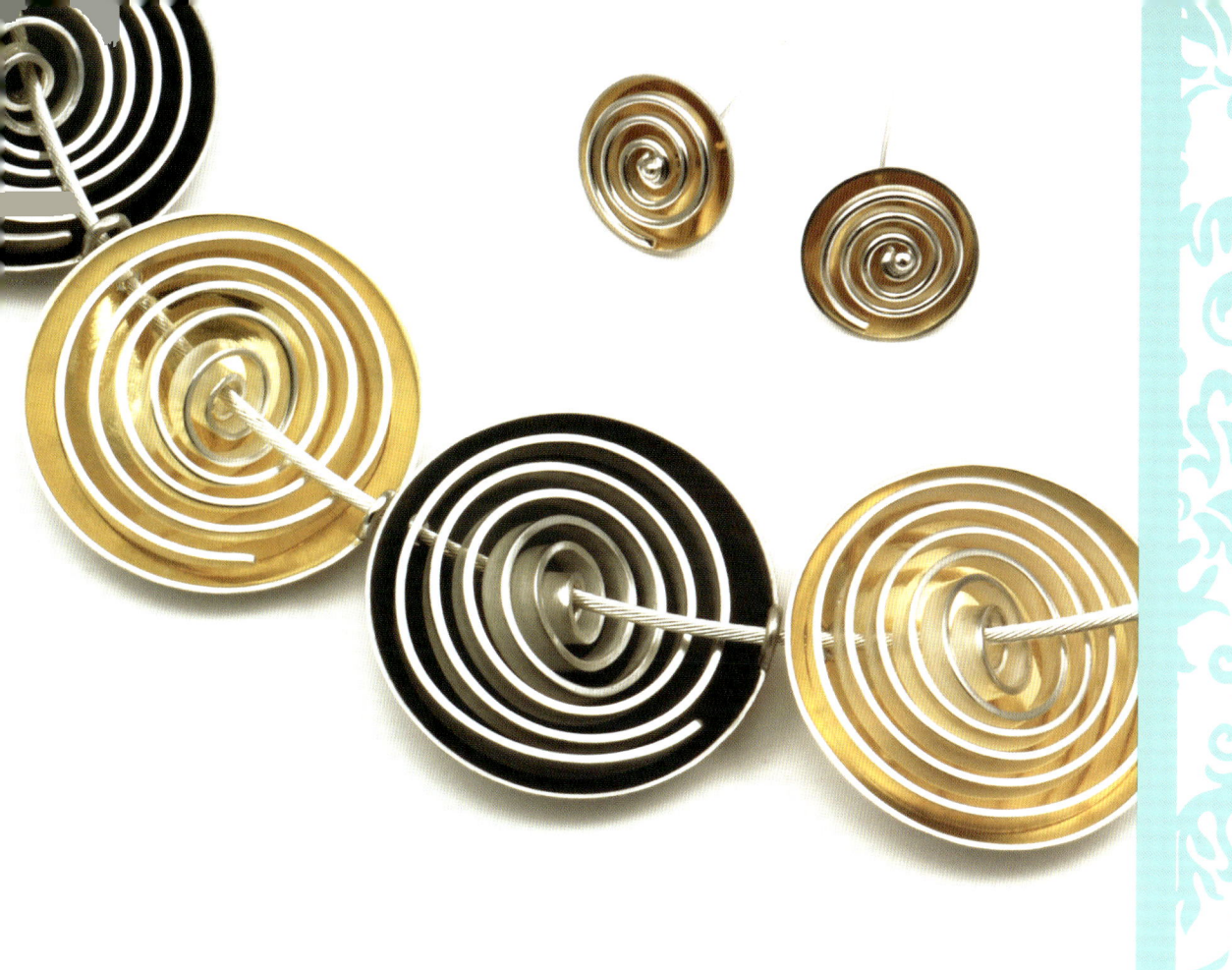

Chapter Eight

Occasions

Does This Look Good On Me?

Occasions

Jewellery is an integral part of the outfit that you are wearing; therefore it is important that it is appropriate for the occasion. The jewellery you wear for work is largely determined by the job that you do. In professional occupations, e.g. lawyers, doctors, accountants, jewellery is required to be minimal. Stud earrings, discreet necklaces or a brooch would be acceptable but flashy rings, jangling bangles, dangly earrings and statement necklaces would not, as they would be seen as distracting and unprofessional. Dangly earrings or a statement necklace would however be appropriate for an evening function.

If you are in a creative industry then very often the normal business dress rules don't apply and the jewellery rules are more liberal. In fact, in some businesses it may even be beneficial to wear statement jewellery. For example, if you were selling jewellery, you would wear your jewellery to generate interest and promote sales (the choice of jewellery that you would wear may depend on where and to whom you are selling).

To be noticed at a special function it may be appropriate to wear a statement piece of jewellery. However, it is important to be aware that less is more– wear only one piece of statement jewellery at a time and keep any other jewellery minimal.

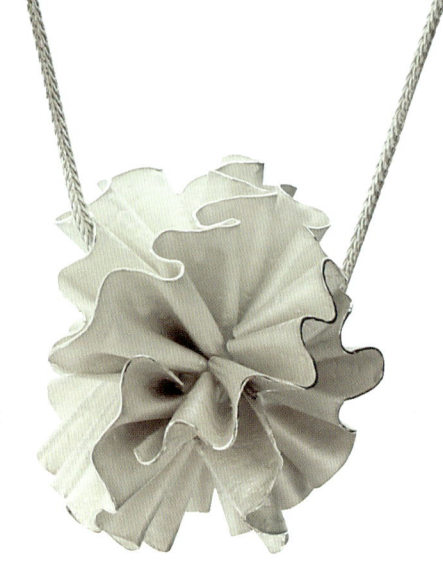

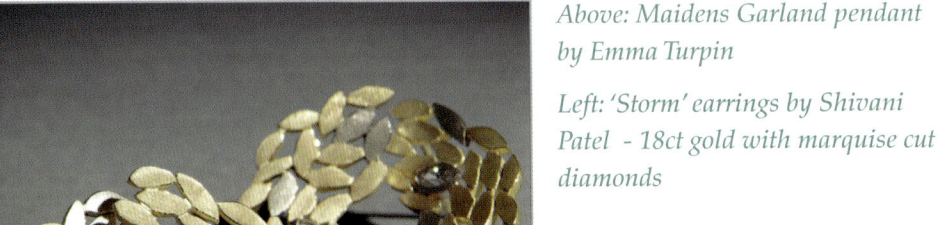

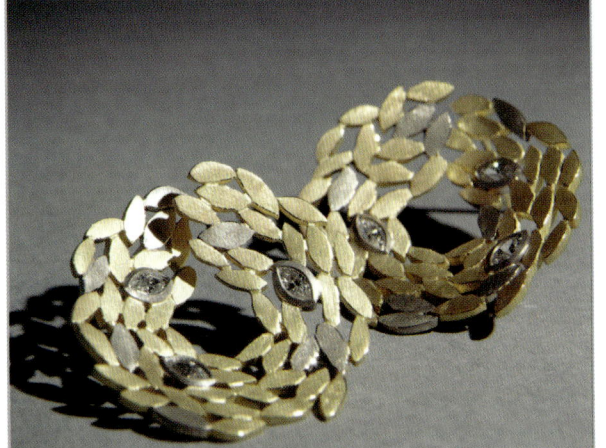

Above: Maidens Garland pendant by Emma Turpin

Left: 'Storm' earrings by Shivani Patel - 18ct gold with marquise cut diamonds

CHAPTER EIGHT: OCCASIONS

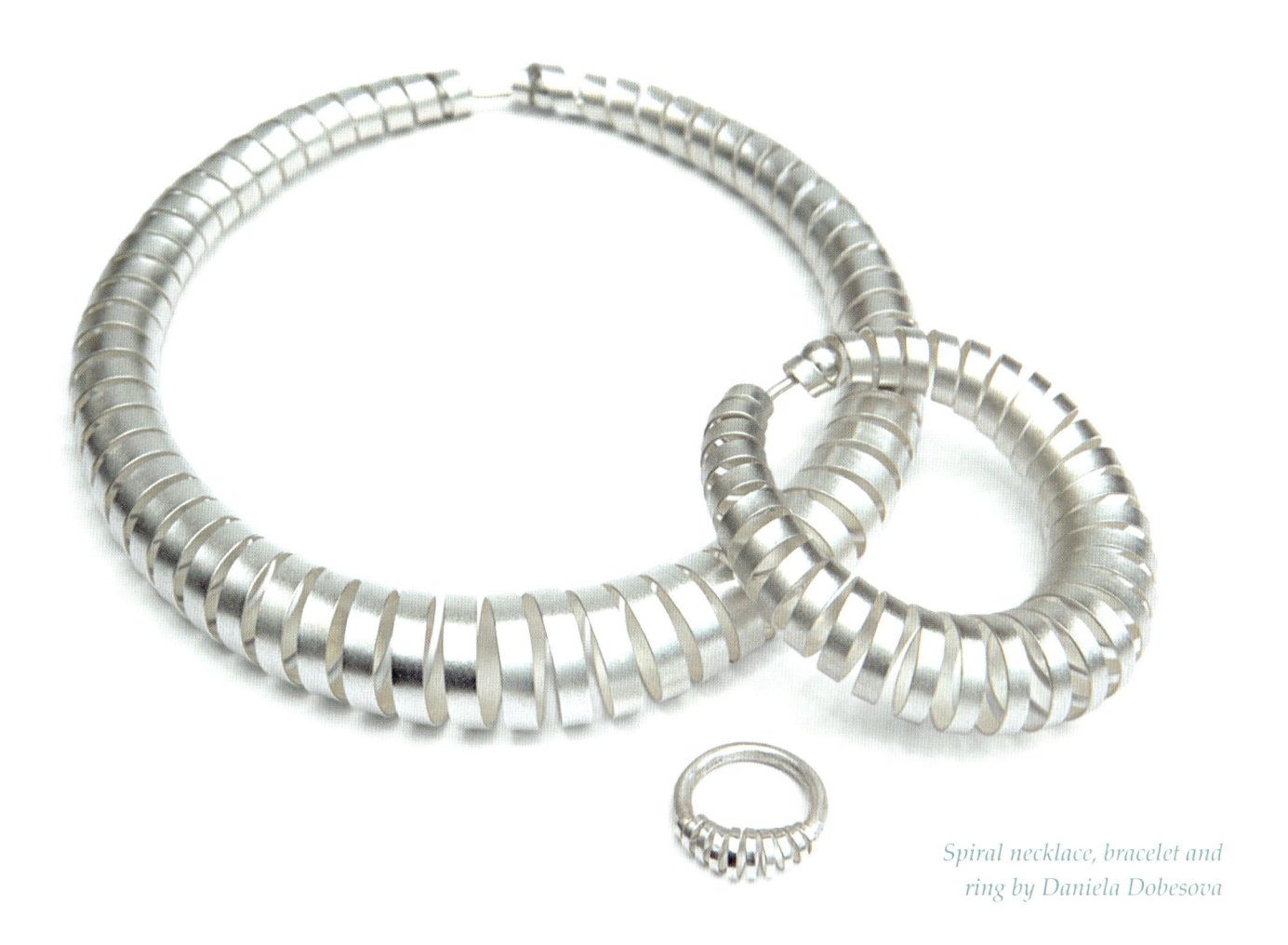

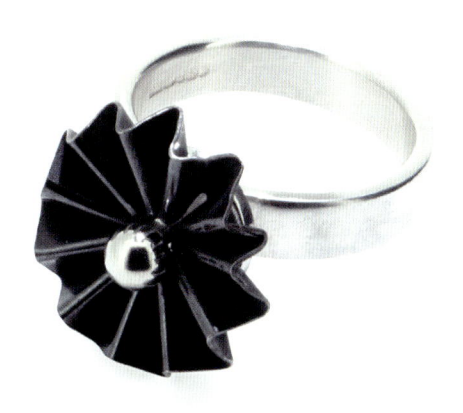

Spiral necklace, bracelet and ring by Daniela Dobesova

Oxidized silver Garland ring by Emma Turpin

If you are attending a race meeting or a wedding and have chosen a hat or fascinator, then avoid also wearing statement earrings and/or necklace as each would draw attention away from the other and the impact of the fabulous hat/fascinator will be spoilt. Should you still want to wear statement jewellery, wear a ring or bracelet, so that it is away from your head.

When you are not limited by work constraints, you have full choice over your jewellery selection. It is still important to follow the basic rules of what suits you, but you are able to express your personality more freely. If you want to wear dangly earrings and a multitude of bangles, then wear them!

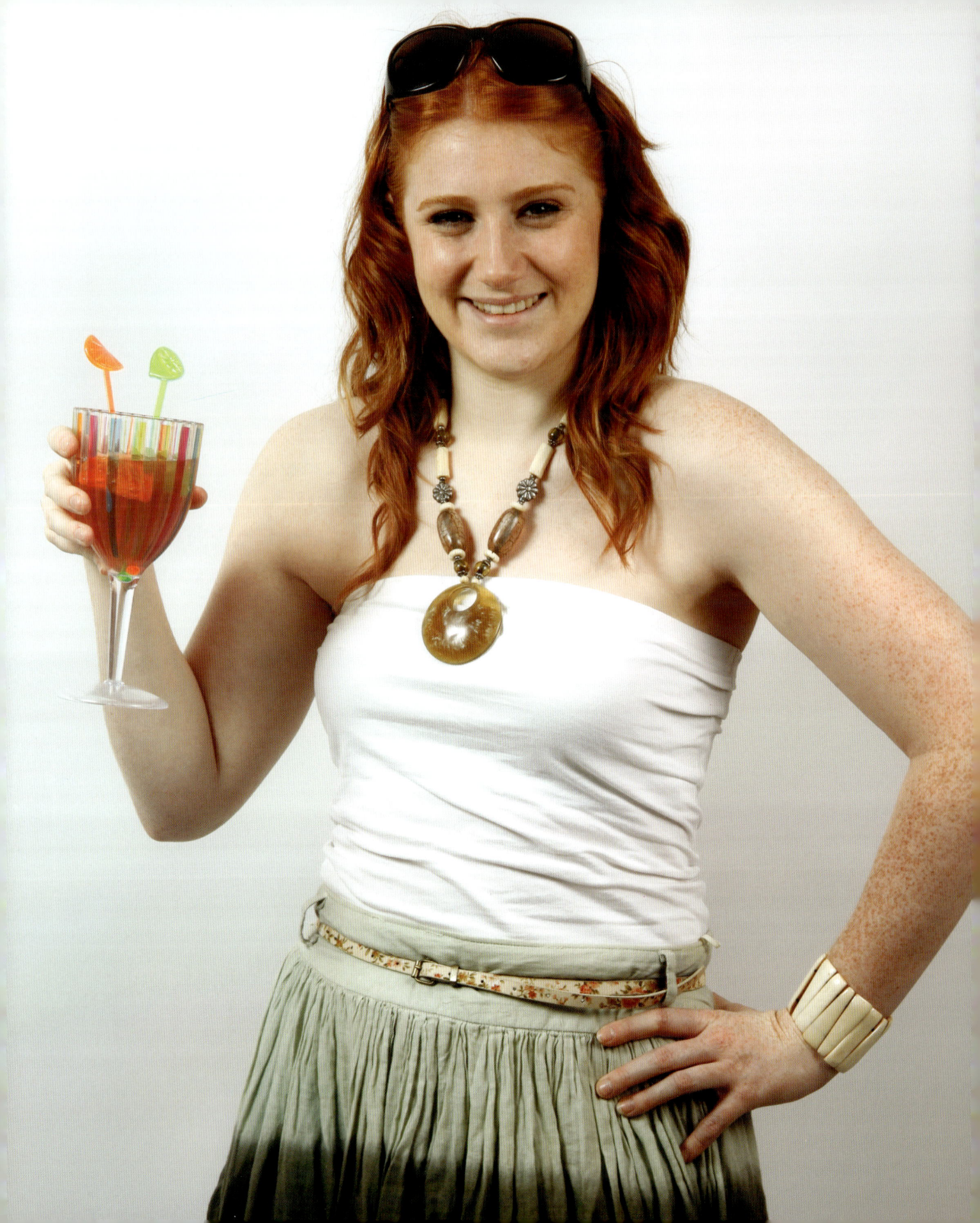

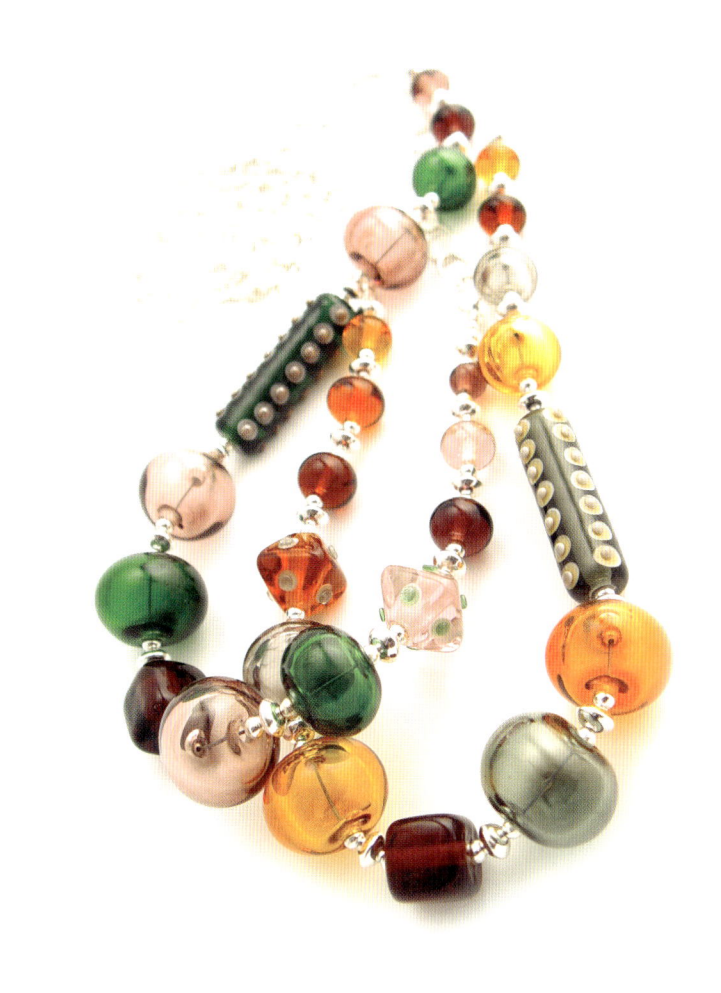

Chapter Nine

Holiday Jewellery

Holiday Jewellery

The annual holiday is something most of us save for, plan and look forward to all year. Holidays offer us a break from our everyday routine and allow us time to recharge and refresh our minds and bodies. Organising our holiday wardrobe is all part of the holiday experience. Jewellery adds the final touch to any given outfit and so should also be included when packing for your holiday.

Holiday jewellery is not necessarily the same as that we would wear normally. Your choice is determined by your destination and the activities you plan while you're away. A city destination will have very different requirements to a beach holiday. The jewellery that is appropriate for a cruise will not be the same as for a skiing break.

There are some basic rules that can be applied when selecting holiday jewellery.

- Leave your high value or sentimental jewellery at home unless it is essential that you take it.

- Select inexpensive items so that should they become lost on the beach or left in a hotel room it would be inconvenient but not devastating.

- Take the minimum number of jewellery pieces possible by carefully selecting versatile items that will compliment a variety of outfits and your physical characteristics.

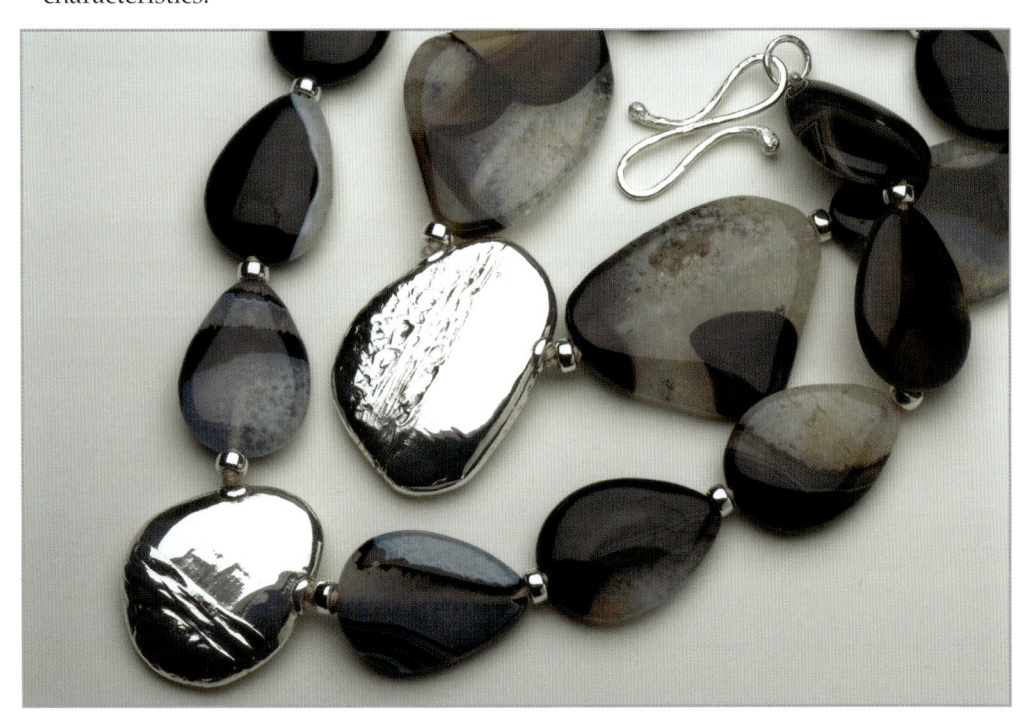

CHAPTER NINE: HOLIDAY JEWELLERY

Beach holiday

This type of holiday really requires minimal jewellery. If you choose plated jewellery note that it may be damaged by either salt or chlorinated water. Jewellery made from wood, shell or glass on cotton cords would be ideal as these are inexpensive and will not be affected by water.

Copper and brass could also be good, if your colours allow. If an aim of your holiday is to obtain a tan, remember that you will get tan lines with jewellery, and so select your pieces carefully to minimize this. A necklace and/or bracelet that compliments your colouring and will generally go with all of your beachwear might be best.

Depending on your venue, you may wish to take additional jewellery for evening wear. Again, a few key pieces that you can wear with several different outfits would be ideal - your own style and personality will determine what you take.

Suggestions for Holiday Jewellery

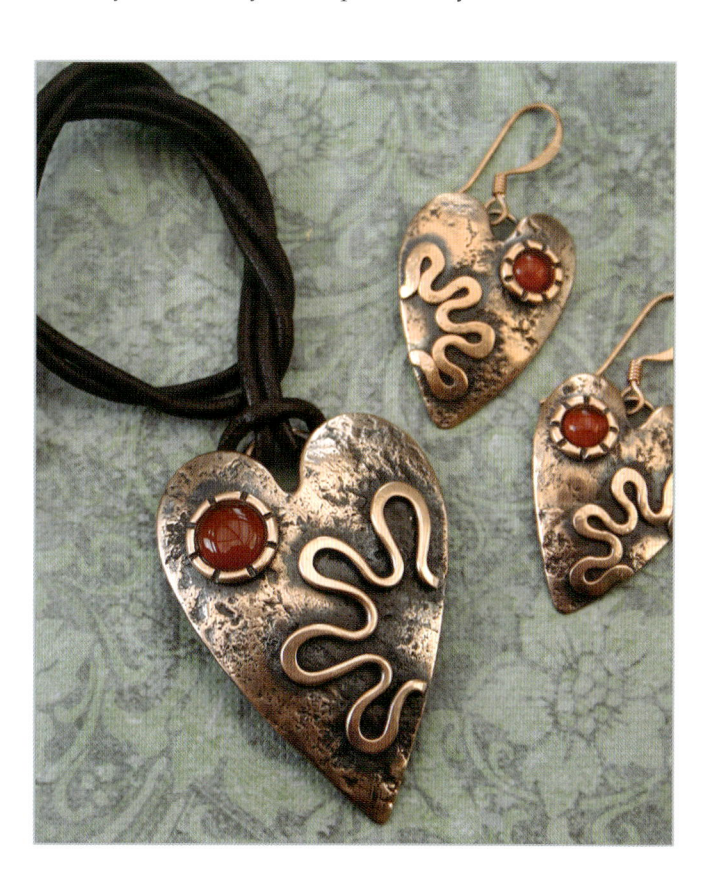

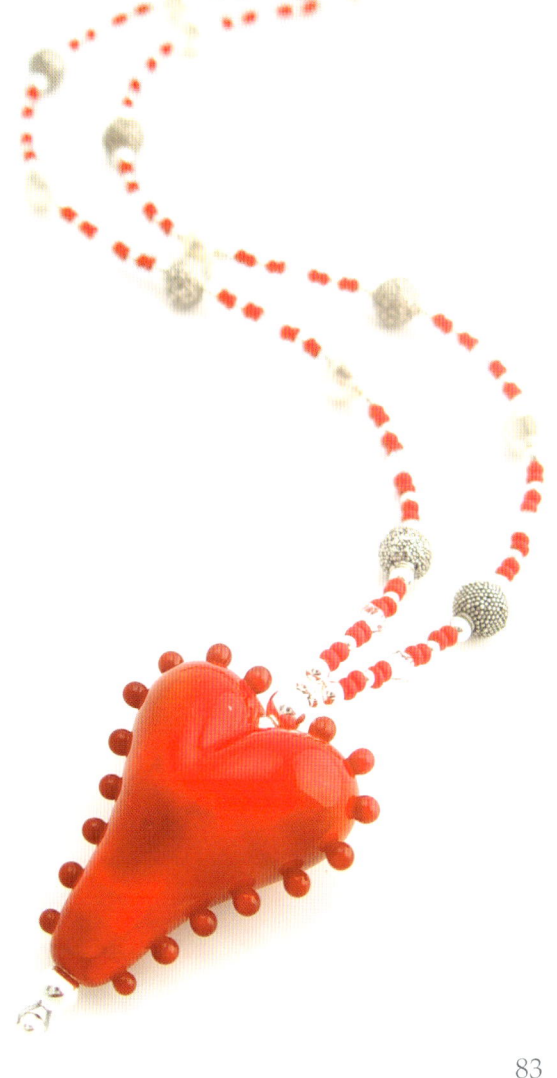

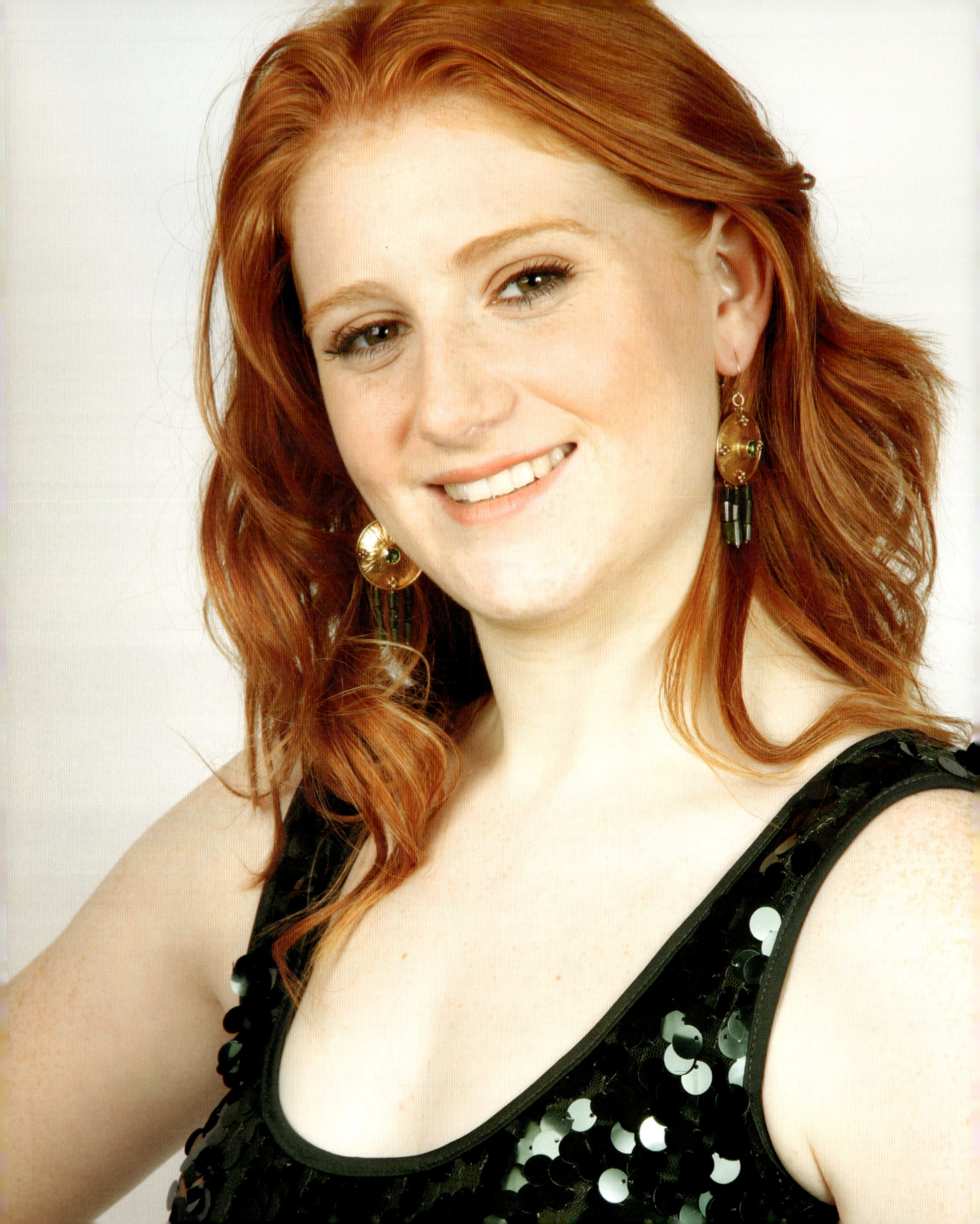

CHAPTER NINE: HOLIDAY JEWELLERY

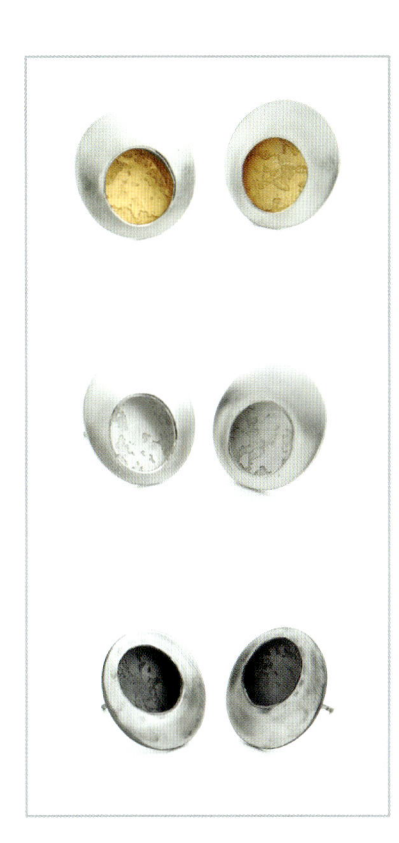

Ski Holiday

On the slopes you will not be able to see any jewellery, so there is little point in wearing any. However, depending on your headwear, a pair of tight fitting stud earrings may be appropriate. For the Après Ski section of your holiday, select versatile pieces that follow the basic rules and can be worn with all of your outfits.

City Break

Jewellery is essential for this type of holiday. It is good to be on trend and chic whilst in a city. Try to restrict the amount of jewellery you take by choosing one pair of earrings, a necklace and a bracelet or ring that will go with everything and then add a pair of drop earrings and possibly an additional necklace for evening wear.

Countryside break

A small selection of jewellery is all that is required. Ideally choose one set of jewellery that can take you through the day into the evening. Your day events will dictate what jewellery is applicable, but possibly a pair of stud earrings, a necklace and a bracelet would be ideal. Statement jewellery is usually not required unless this is your personality type, or you have a special dinner planned.

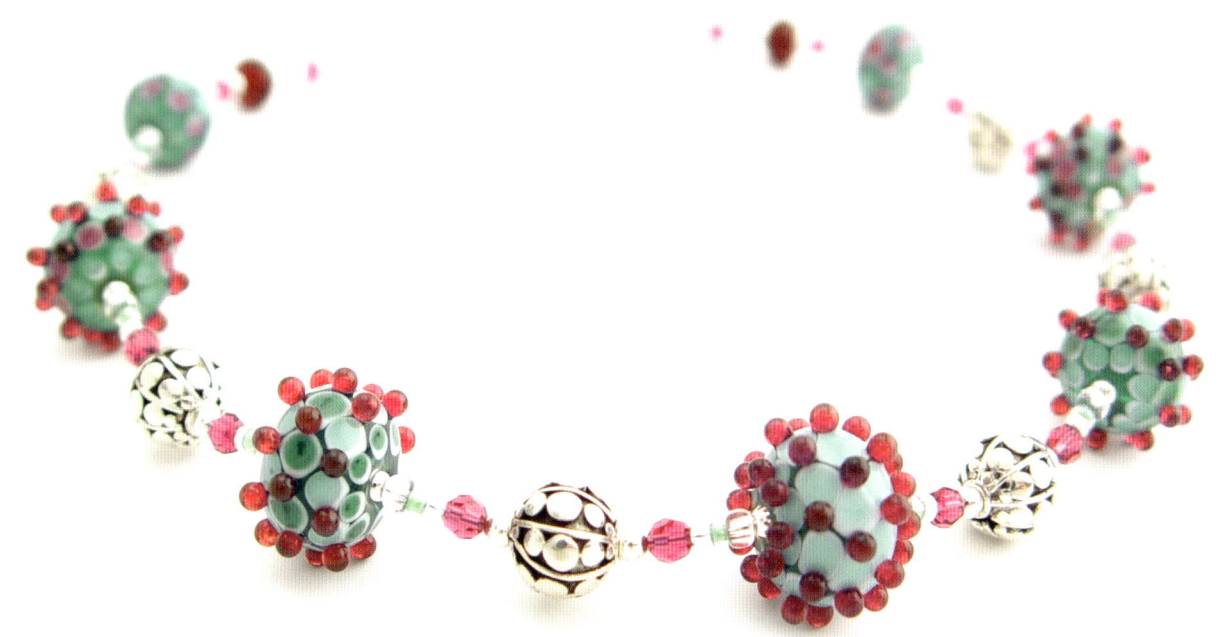

85

Cruise

You will probably wear more jewellery on this type of holiday than you will on any other. Your daytime attire will depend largely on what the planned activities are on that day and where you are in the world.

If you will be lounging around a pool then select items that will not be affected by chlorinated or sea water. If you are visiting a city then a pair of stud earrings, necklace and/or bracelet appropriate for your physical characteristics and personality would be ideal.

On a cruise ship it is usual to dress for dinner; evening dress is often necessary. Statement jewellery is ideal for evening wear, so take a small selection that allows some variety over your vacation.

Selecting a collection that 'goes together' and that can be 'mixed and matched' works well. One evening you may choose a statement neck piece (necklace, collar or torque), a pair of stud earrings and a dress ring and on another evening dangly earrings and a bracelet.

Remember, to make a positive impact, don't wear too many statement pieces or else the effect will be minimized. It may be possible to choose a statement necklace that can be varied e.g. a pendant that can slide over different pearls or beads to change the look; designer/makers can often offer this option.

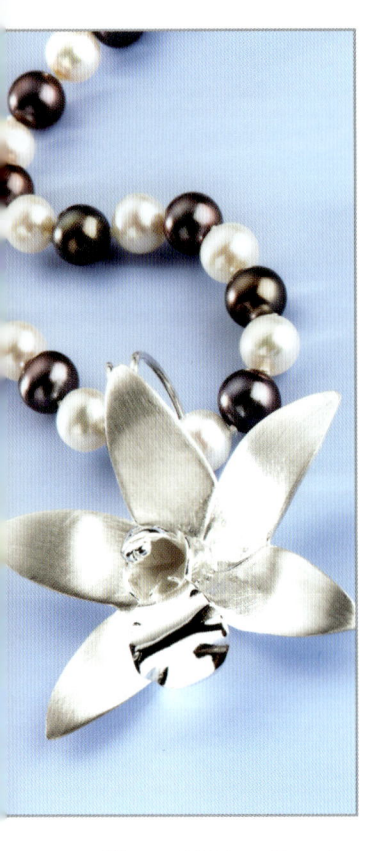

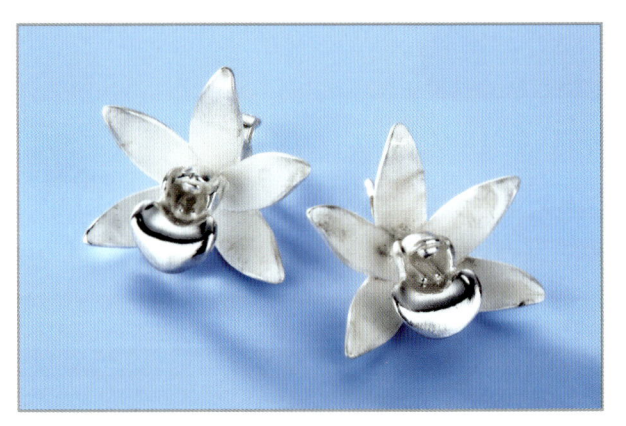

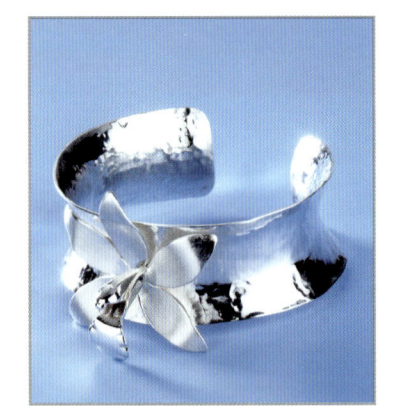

The orchid jewellery is perfect for the evening. The pendant can be worn with different pearls or beads. No necklace is required if you wear the cuff with the earrings.

Adventure break

General advice here is to leave your jewellery at home. All jewellery can be a hazard on an activity-based holiday, so it is better not to wear any. A minimal collection may be required for the evenings depending on your itinerary.

CHAPTER NINE: HOLIDAY JEWELLERY

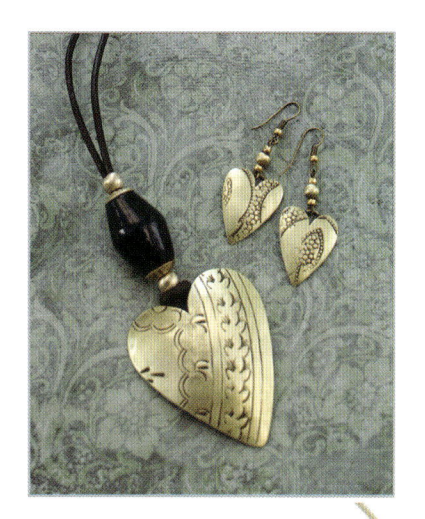

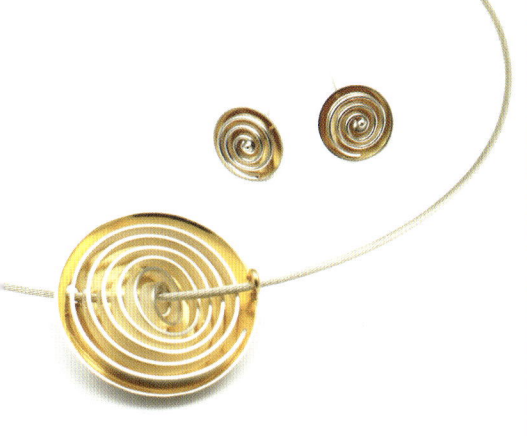

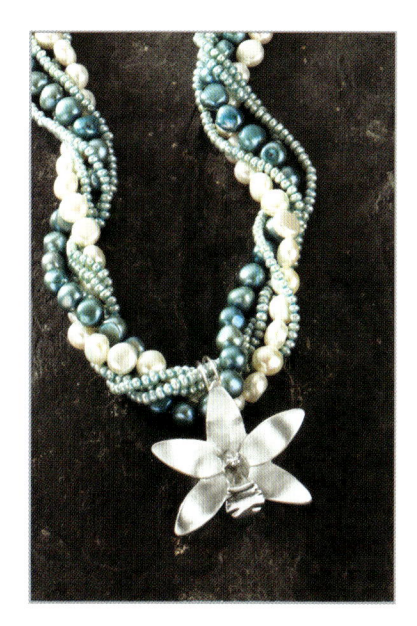

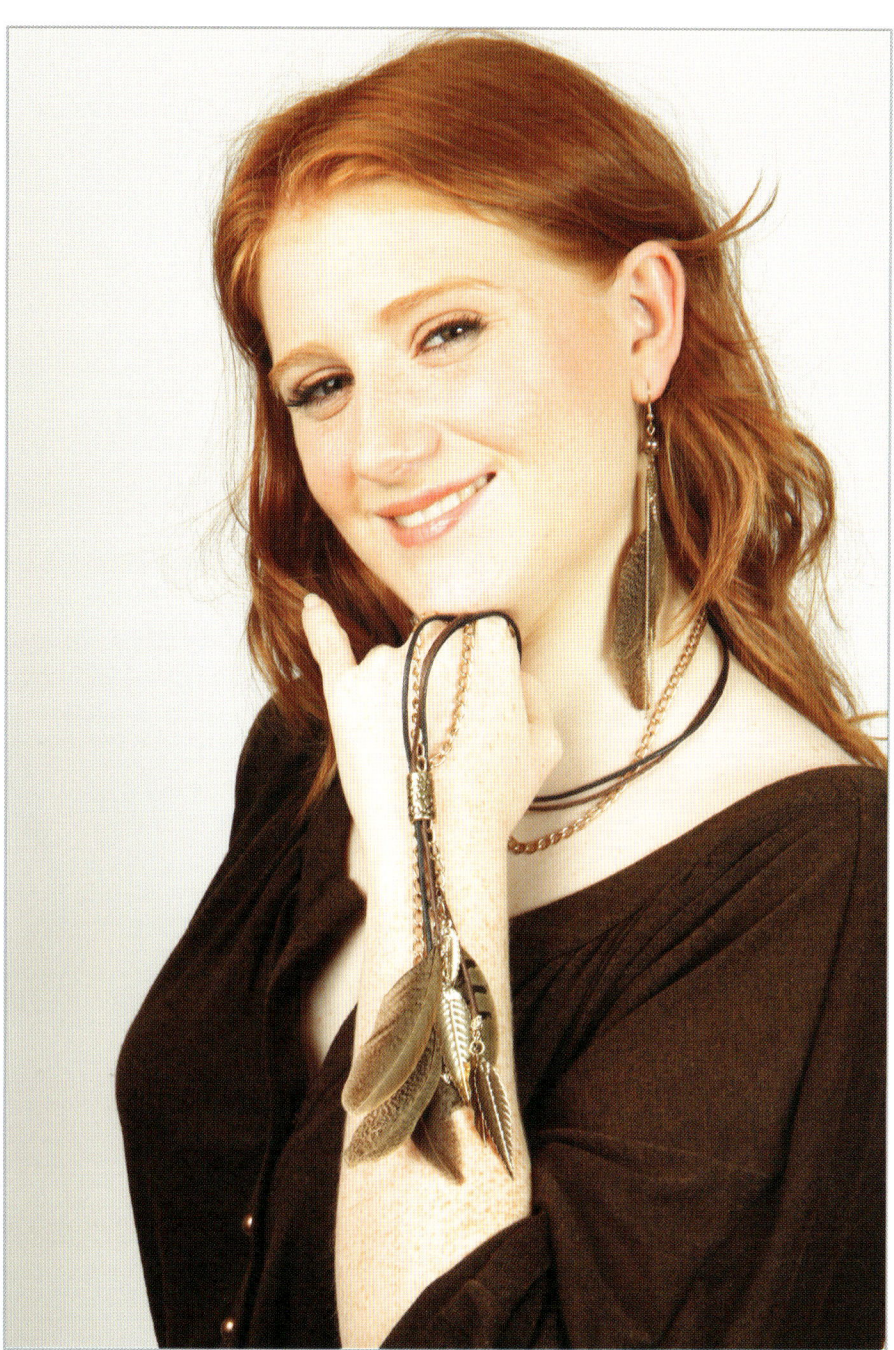

Inexpensive, fun fashion jewellery is perfect to take on holiday

87

Eternity pendants by KFD Jewellery

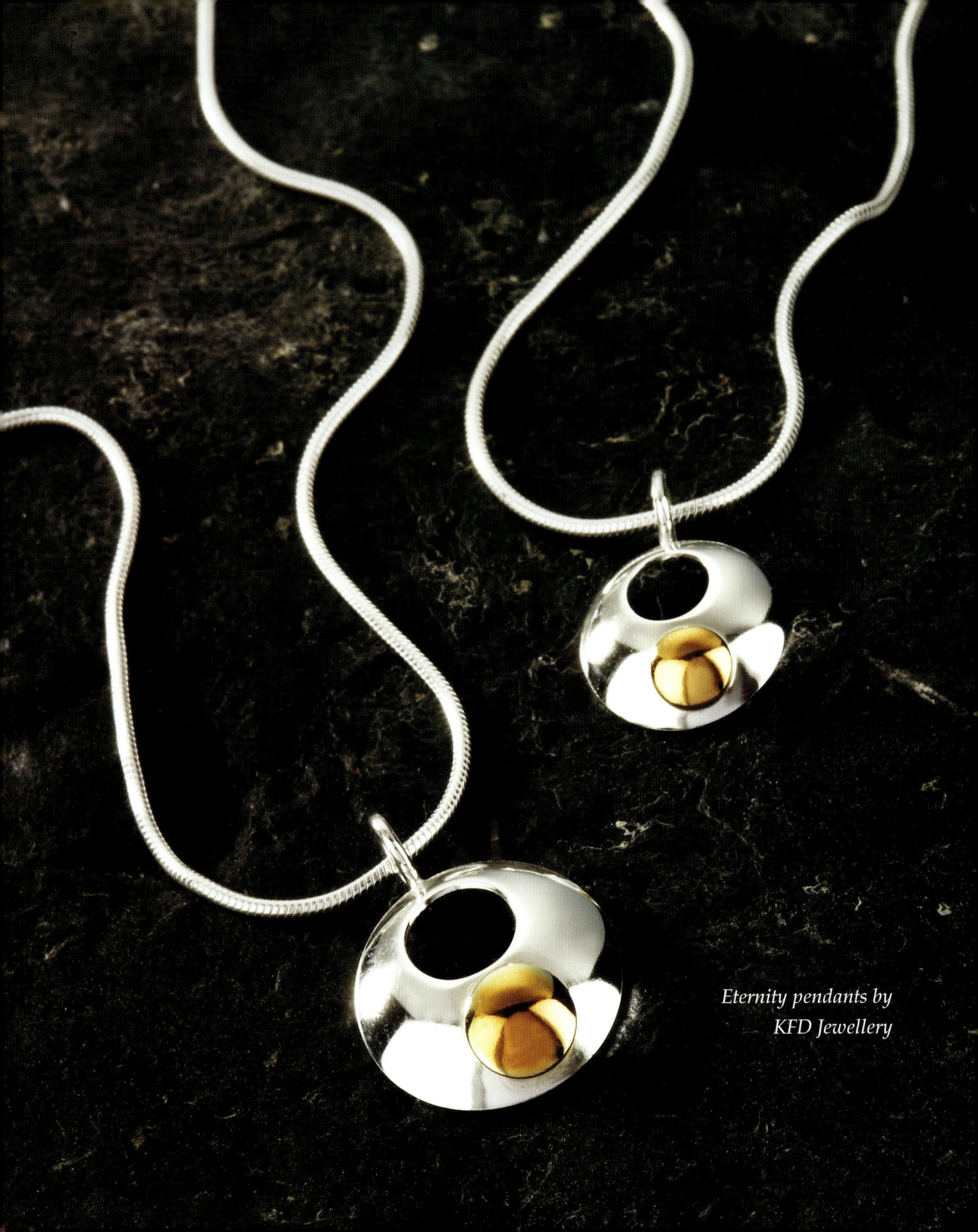

CHAPTER TEN
About the Designers

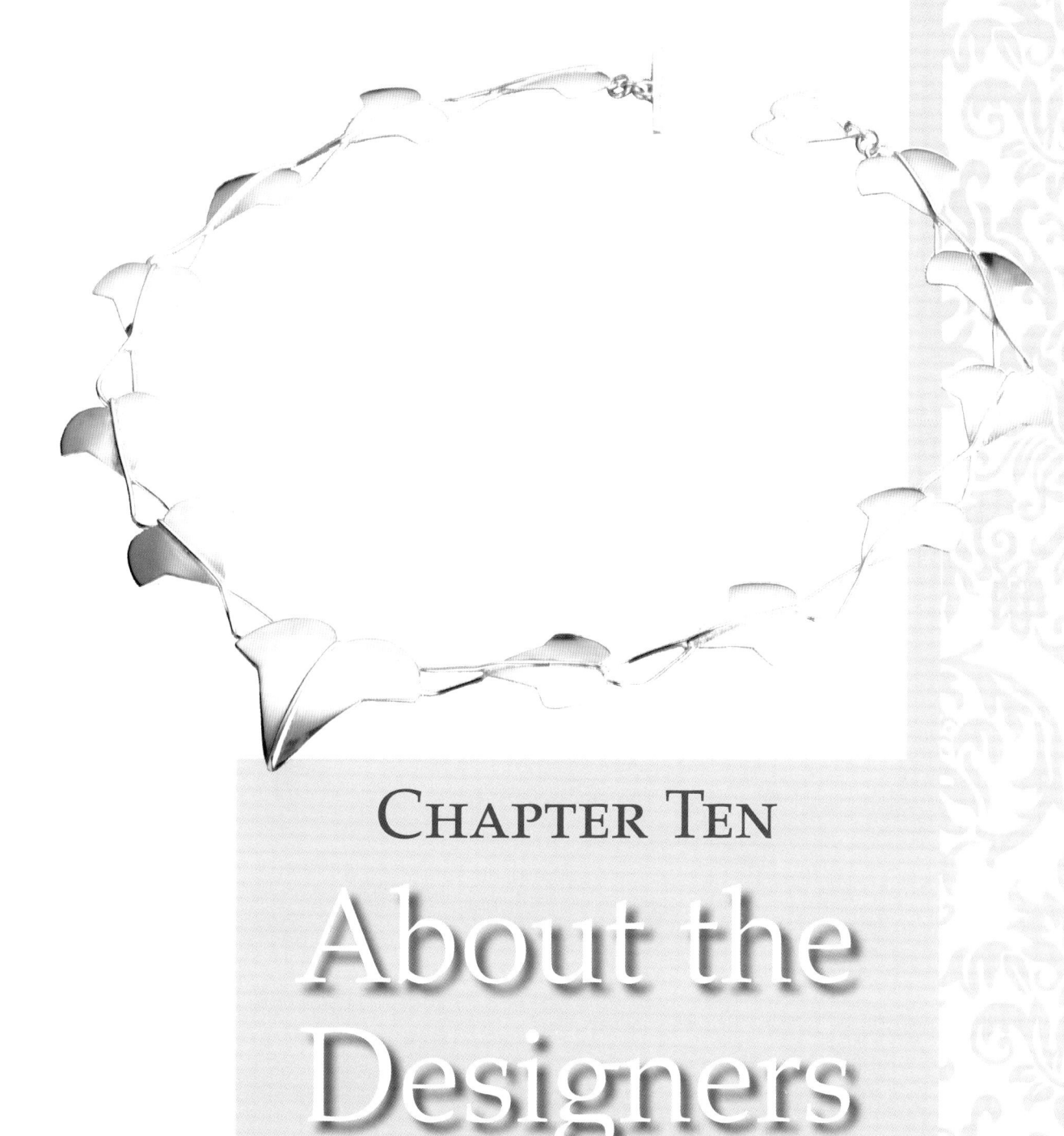

All of the designer/makers featured in this book are based in the UK.

Does This Look Good On Me?

Carole Allen

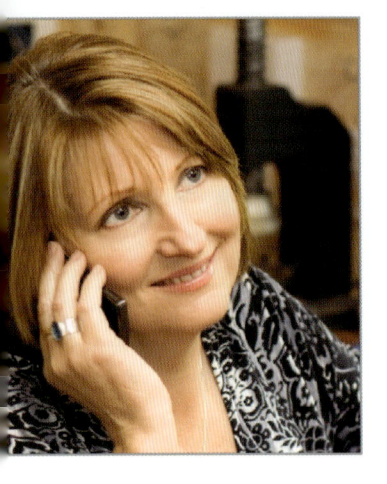

Carole began her career making handmade jewellery in the early 1990s. She added to her skills by taking master classes at a selection of prestigious establishments such as West Dean College and the School of Jewellery at Birmingham University.

Carole designs and makes handcrafted jewellery in her studio in Cornwall. Her designs are inspired by the Cornish seascapes and the colourful flowers in her environment. Her jewellery is wearable, feminine and affordable. In addition to the traditional silver and gold jewellery, Carole has developed a range of brightly coloured aluminum jewellery and more recently added coloured acrylics to her portfolio.

In 2008 Carole opened a new purpose-built studio on the periphery of Camborne and now offers jewellery classes to share her skills and knowledge.

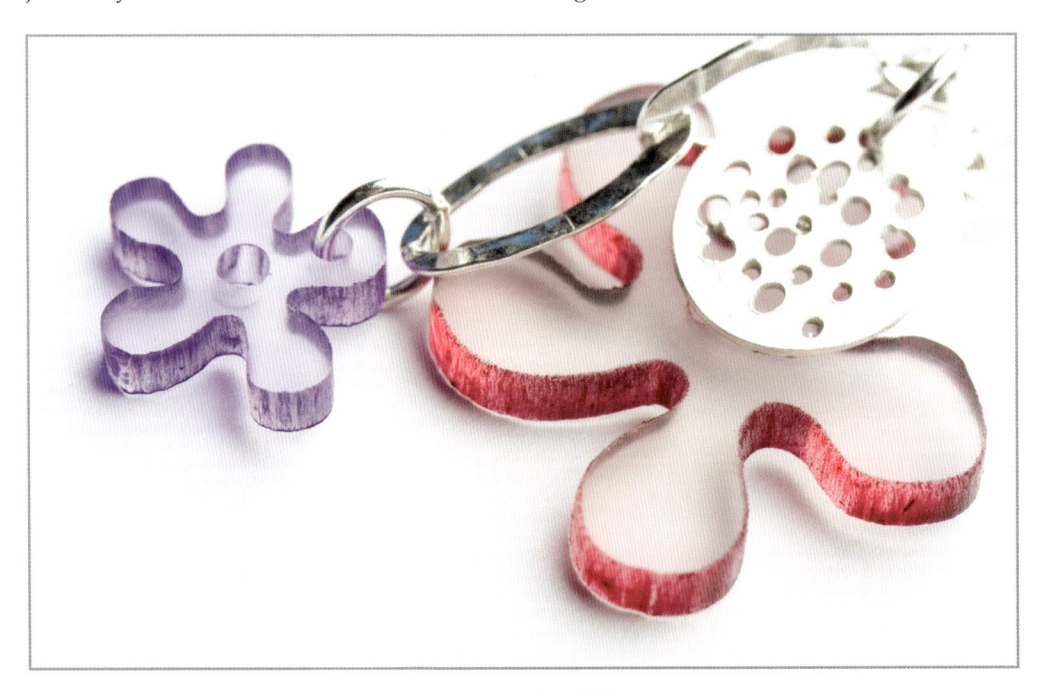

www.caroleallenjewellery.co.uk
contact@caroleallenjewellery.co.uk
+44(0)1209715605
+44(0)7810770219

CHAPTER TEN: ABOUT THE DESIGNERS

Lyn Antley

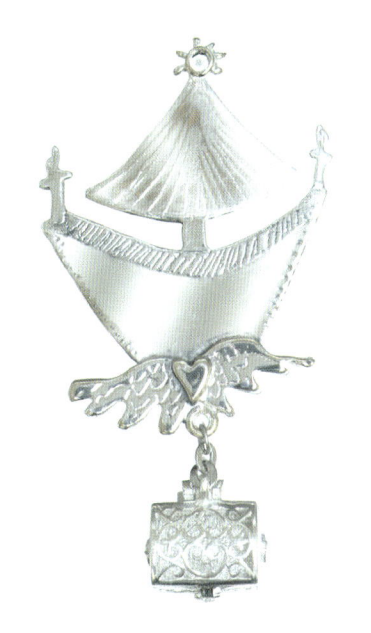

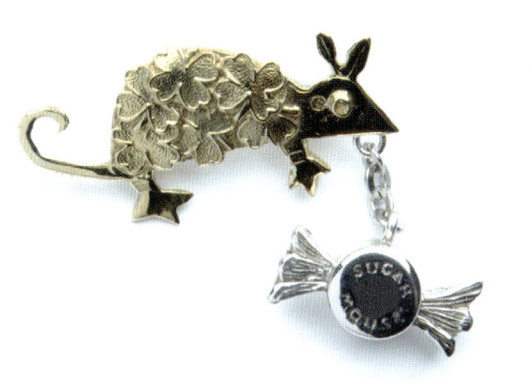

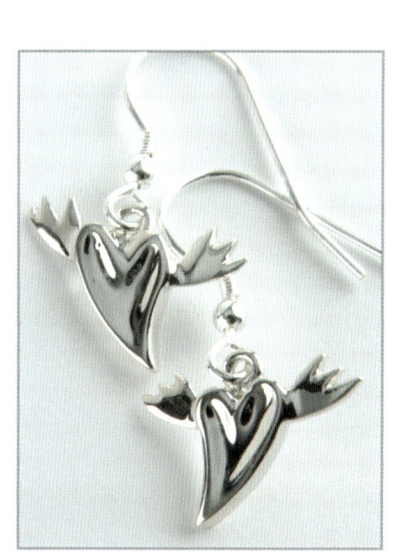

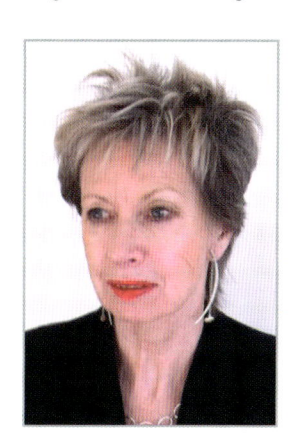

Lyn went to art school with the intention of becoming a textile designer, but, after taking a jewellery course, she knew that she wanted to work with metal and design jewellery. Lyn uses a combination of silver, gold and brass to make witty jewellery with personality and imagination. Her jewellery designs are inspired both by her travels to faraway places and by the fairy stories she has read to her children. The creatures Lyn observes from her Worcester home also have been a source of inspiration, leading to the creation of whimsical brooches such as 'naughty fox' and 'dancing hare'.

Many of Lyn's customers are avid collectors of her work and purchase her new pieces as soon as they are available. Some pieces are like metal toys with moving parts, whilst others have 'secret' images and inscriptions on the reverse.

When asked about the type of person who buys her work Lyn replied:

"My customers generally are people who like something out of the ordinary; like each item to have a story or a provenance; like items that are fun and witty. They generally are extroverts, people who like their jewellery to be noticed as they want to be noticed, such as actresses, teachers, TV personalities, confident people who know their own mind."

Lyn has a studio in Birmingham's Jewellery Quarter and sells her work through galleries, museums, shops and fairs. Her work has been sold to customers in North America, South Africa, Australia and Germany.

www.lynantley.co.uk
sales@lynantley.co.uk
+44(0)1215511414

91

Does This Look Good On Me?

Daniela Dobesova

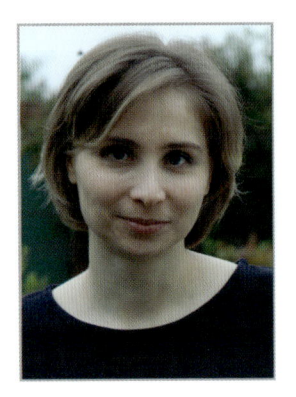

The award-winning Daniela Dobesova started her training in her home city of Prague at The College of Art & Design. She continued her training at Richmond College of Art in London, graduating in 2003.

Daniela has developed a series of coiling and wire forming techniques that are truly innovative.

"I use a range of wire forming and self-developed coiling techniques, combined with traditional skills, to create distinctive and elegant jewellery, with the emphasis placed on the quality of the craftsmanship and originality of design. With their classic feel, their clean lines and symmetry, all pieces are highly wearable, some more appropriate as everyday wear and others for special occasions.

The jewellery appeals to those who take a genuine interest in original design and seek to differentiate themselves by making a statement of personal choice. For some this personal choice is expressed through the boldness of the one-off statement pieces, while for others it is achieved in a more subtle way by selecting pieces expressing classical elegance."

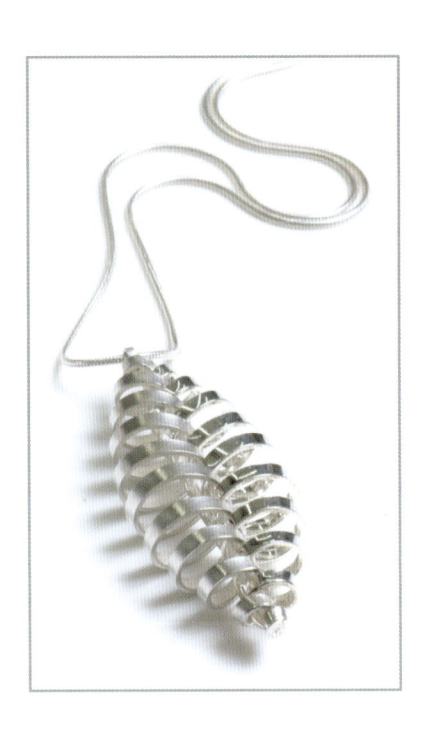

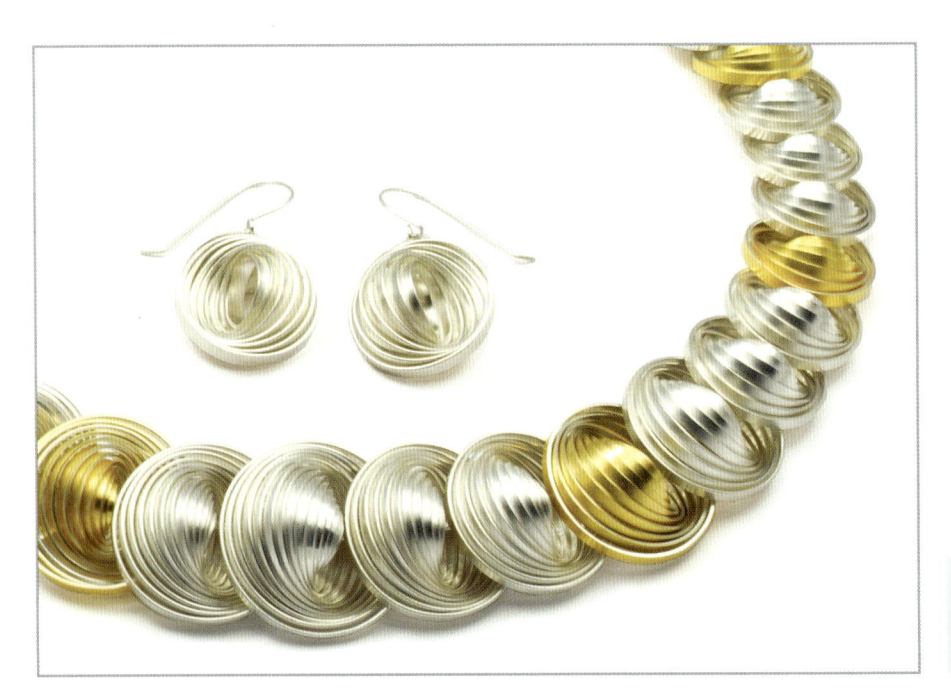

www.danieladobesova.com
daniela@danieladobesova.com
+44(0)1344291888

CHAPTER TEN: ABOUT THE DESIGNERS

Karen Faulkner-Dunkley

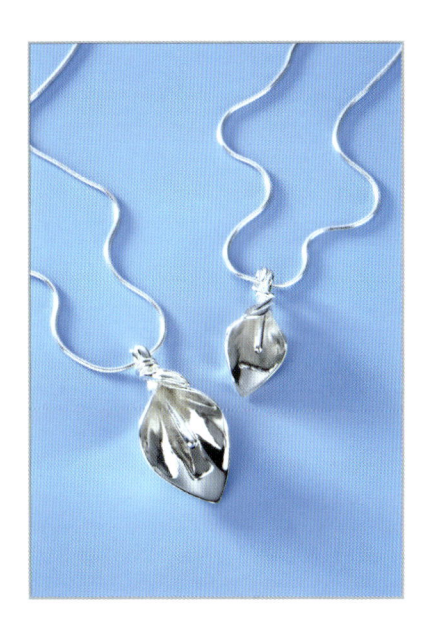

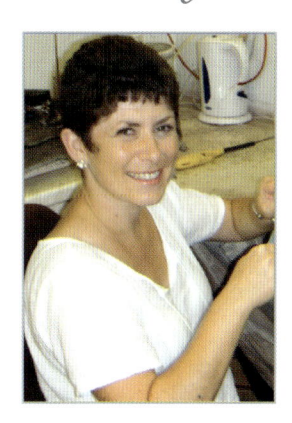

As a lecturer in the 1990s I was always referred to as KFD, therefore when I began making jewellery the name KFD Jewellery was an obvious choice.

When designing my jewellery I often produce rough sketches of my thoughts which I then develop into paper models to see if my ideas will 'work' as jewellery. I visualize in 3D rather than 2D, so I find that a paper model gives me a better idea of what the finished jewellery will look like.

Once I have made any alterations to the paper model, I create the jewellery in metal from silver sheet and wire. Texture is important in my designs, with a variety of finishes being employed in each jewellery collection.

Often my jewellery consists of a mixture of silver and gold as I find that this tends to suit more people. I also produce jewellery in ranges with a variety of pieces in different sizes, so that there is something to suit and fit every individual in every range.

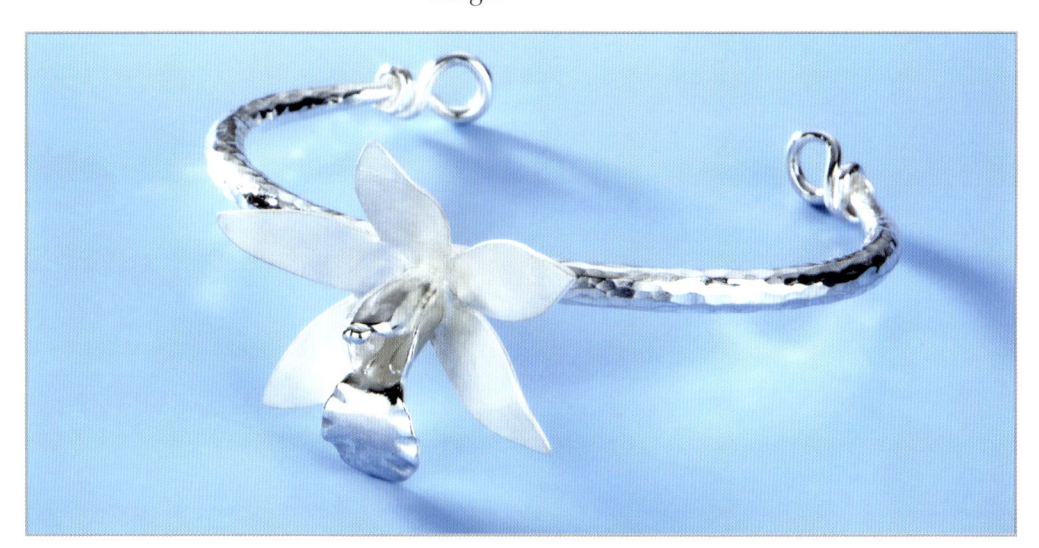

www.kfdjewellery.co.uk
www.kfdjewelery.com
karen@kfdjewellery.co.uk
+44(0)7947113359

Does This Look Good On Me?

Theresa Galanides

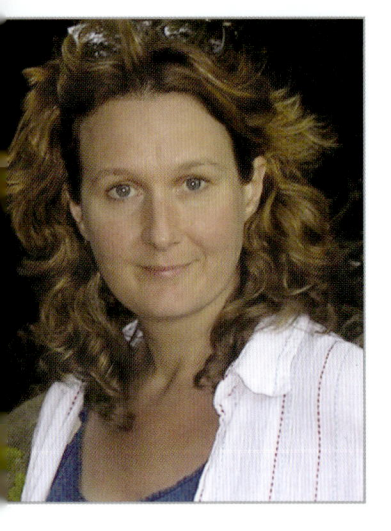

Theresa Galanides trained in 3 dimensional glass design at Lancashire Polytechnic, graduating in 1991. She won the British Artists in Glass - Student of the Year award that year and with the prize money bought a collection of jewellery-making tools and taught herself basic jewellery-making techniques.

She always had a love of jewellery and developed an interest in working with recycled materials. Her first exhibition was at the Ancient High House in her home town of Stafford. This led to taking the step to professional jeweller in 1994. Since then Theresa has taken part in exhibitions all over the country. Her main focus is on Art and Design events in the UK and on commissioned work.

Theresa designs and makes affordable jewellery in copper and brass. Semiprecious stones are used with some designs.

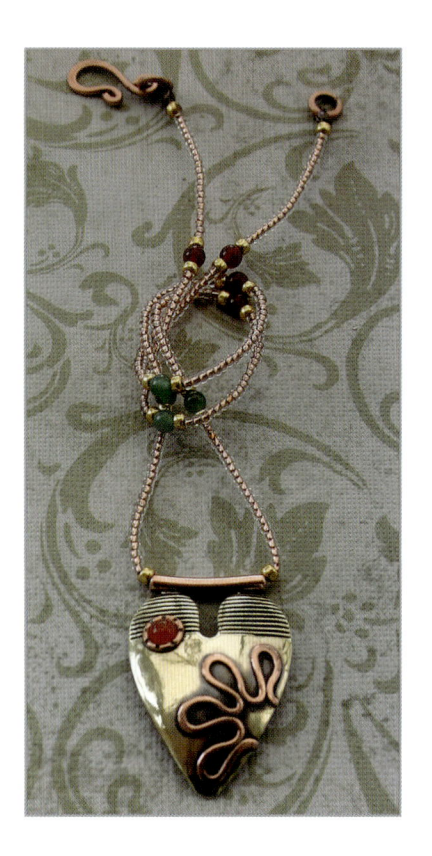

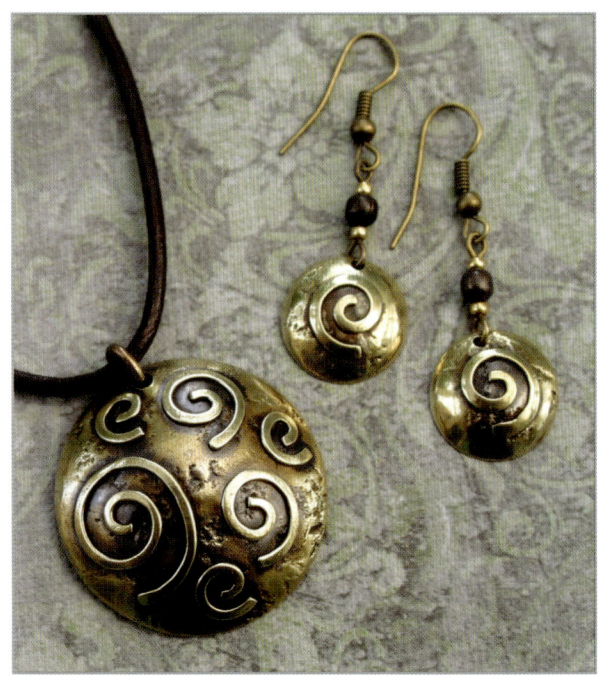

www.theresagalanides.com
neat@galanides.wanadoo.co.uk

CHAPTER TEN: ABOUT THE DESIGNERS

Rachel Gogerly graduated with a BA honours degree in 1986, which included studying for a year in one of London's leading enamel studios where she was classically trained in the fine techniques and finishing processes of champlevé basse taille and guilloché.

This award-winning designer maker of contemporary silver and enamel jewellery has attracted numerous awards including those from The Platinum Corporation and The Goldsmiths' Craft Council. She has undertaken a number of major commissions from patrons including The Lord Mayor of York and The Worshipful Company of Goldsmiths.

Rachel Gogerly is a member of The Guild of Enamellers and British Society of Enamellers. In 2002 Rachel became a Freeman of the Worshipful Company of Goldsmiths.

As a leading contemporary designer and expert in her field, Rachel has lectured on the techniques of fine enamelling and taught jewellery and enamelling extensively.

She exhibits her work widely in the UK. She is a regular exhibitor at many well-established, prestigious shows. Rachel receives regular press and media coverage, locally and nationally.

She talks about her work with passion:

"I work with transparent enamels because I love the qualities – they have a real vibrancy within the colour, which comes from the fact they are created from metal oxides. The clarity of colour also gives the enamel depth and life, as the enamel is so reflective. These two elements make the enamel very eye catching.

It is this vibrancy and clarity that makes the enamel so appealing to the wearer too, because it makes the colours easy to wear as they pick up the colours around them. Any colour that suits the skin tone of that person will actually go with anything they wear and some of the enamel colours almost appear to change colour when put against different fabrics. It is one of the things my customers regularly comment on, that they can wear their pieces with so many different things and they give both the outfit and the wearer a real 'lift'."

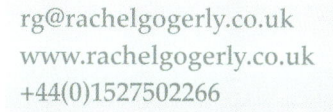

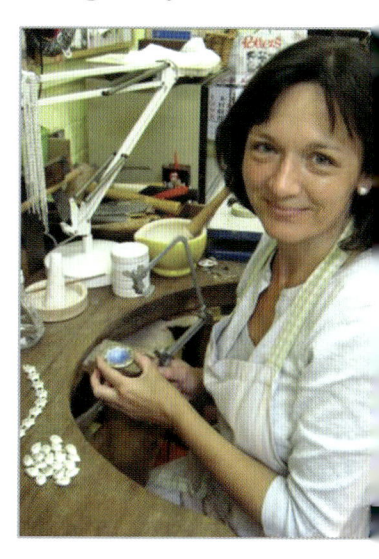

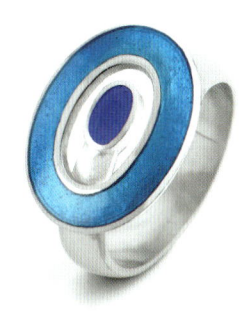

Rachel Gogerly

rg@rachelgogerly.co.uk
www.rachelgogerly.co.uk
+44(0)1527502266

DOES THIS LOOK GOOD ON ME?

Simone Micallef

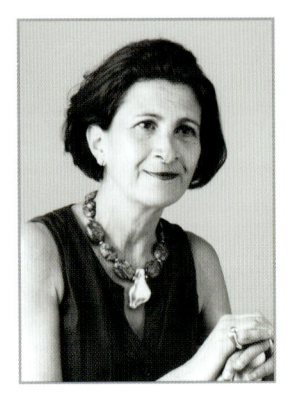

Previously a midwife in her home nation of Malta, the award-winning Simone Micallef re-trained to become a jeweller at Central St Martins, London.

Simone Micallef designs unique necklaces and other jewellery from her London workshop. The semiprecious stone beads are her starting point: she skillfully designs metal shapes to reflect and compliment the chosen beads. Metal and stone are then combined synergistically in the necklace to produce a piece in harmony.

Simone Micallef understands the need to match the necklace to the wearer in its colour, size and form. She believes in *"empowering women by helping them choose a piece that enhances their own natural beauty, picking on their qualities, features and character so that the piece adds kudos without overpowering. I aim to continue to find good homes for my pieces and to give this personalized customer care, advice and satisfaction. This is the true reward for my art."*

Each piece of jewellery that Simone creates is bespoke. Like a well loved cashmere sweater it is designed to be worn with anything, anywhere. Simone explains "my necklaces can be worn during the day to go shopping or to quickly dress up a jeans and T-shirt outfit to go out for dinner."

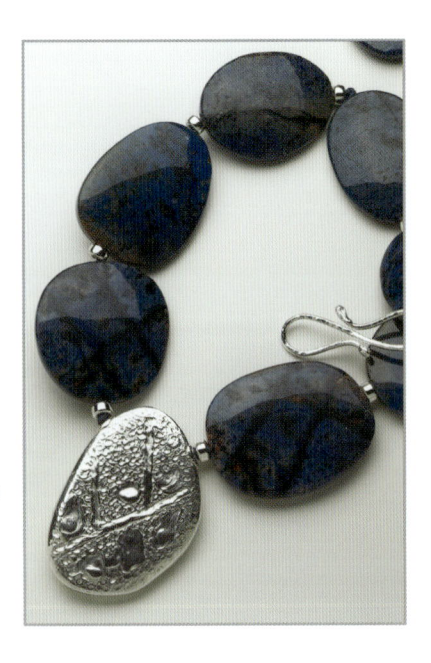

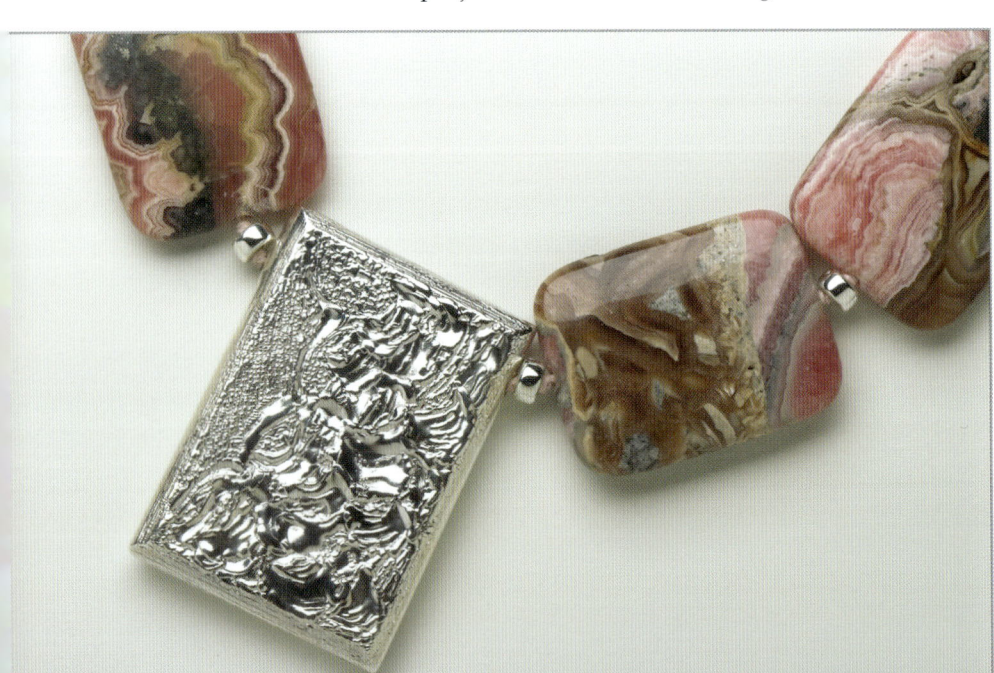

www.simonemicallef.com
simone@simonemicallef.com
+44(0)2084441340
+44(0)7946600467

CHAPTER TEN: ABOUT THE DESIGNERS

Shivani Patel

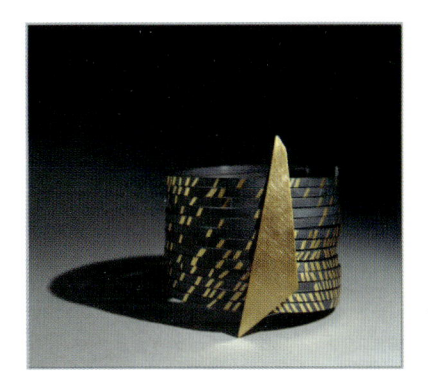

The award-winning Shivani Patel graduated from the The School of Jewellery, Birmingham University in 2005 with a 1st class BA (Hons) in Silversmithing. Since graduating Shivani has opened her own studio in Worcester, to showcase her work. She specialises in the design and construction of individual handmade pieces of jewellery.

"My collection of work centres around dramatic one-off pieces of jewellery. Although each piece may be large in size, surfaces are delicately textured and the designs are highly refined. The colour pallets I work with are pure rich gold combined with deep charcoal patinated silver and coloured gemstones. These pieces would suit a wearer that likes to dress in stylish, simple, tailored and sculptural outfits with clean lines. Combining textures and block colours within clothing is also complimentary as excessive pattern and colour can work against the overall look.

My pieces are easy to wear for a person of any colouring, as colours within the jewellery are minimal and flattering. I encourage buyers of my statement pieces to wear them often and not be afraid. These pieces are made to be worn and they can transform simple day and evening wear looks. Each piece should be worn with confidence."

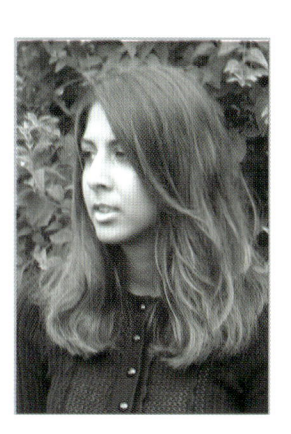

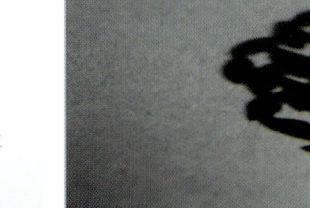

Shivani Patel
mail@shivanijewellery.co.uk
www.shivanijewellery.co.uk
+44(0)7779115080

Does This Look Good On Me?

Heather Stowell

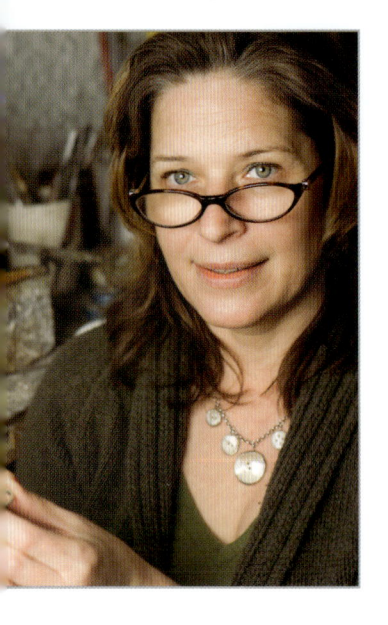

Heather graduated from the Guildhall University of London (Sir John Cass) in 1989 with a BA (Hons) degree in jewellery and silversmithing. She established her own workshop in Clerkenwell, London, supplying galleries in the UK, New York and Tokyo. Now relocated in Cambridgeshire, Heather has developed a new popular range of jewellery inspired by her love of old buttons. She lovingly selects old buttons made from a range of materials such as mother of pearl, glass and enamel and transforms them into eye-catching contemporary jewellery. The buttons are set in sterling silver, preserved for future generations.

Heather says, *"I love to work to commission, setting clients' own buttons, to make a special family piece, or a keepsake, or to create a truly personal gift for a birthday, christening or wedding."*

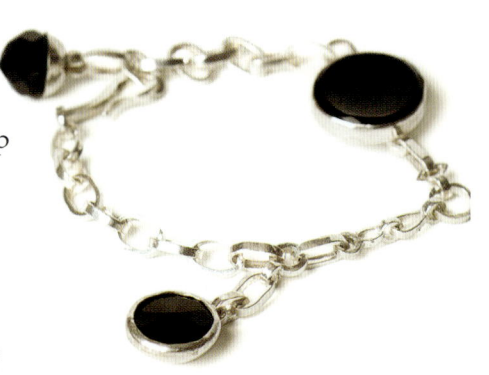

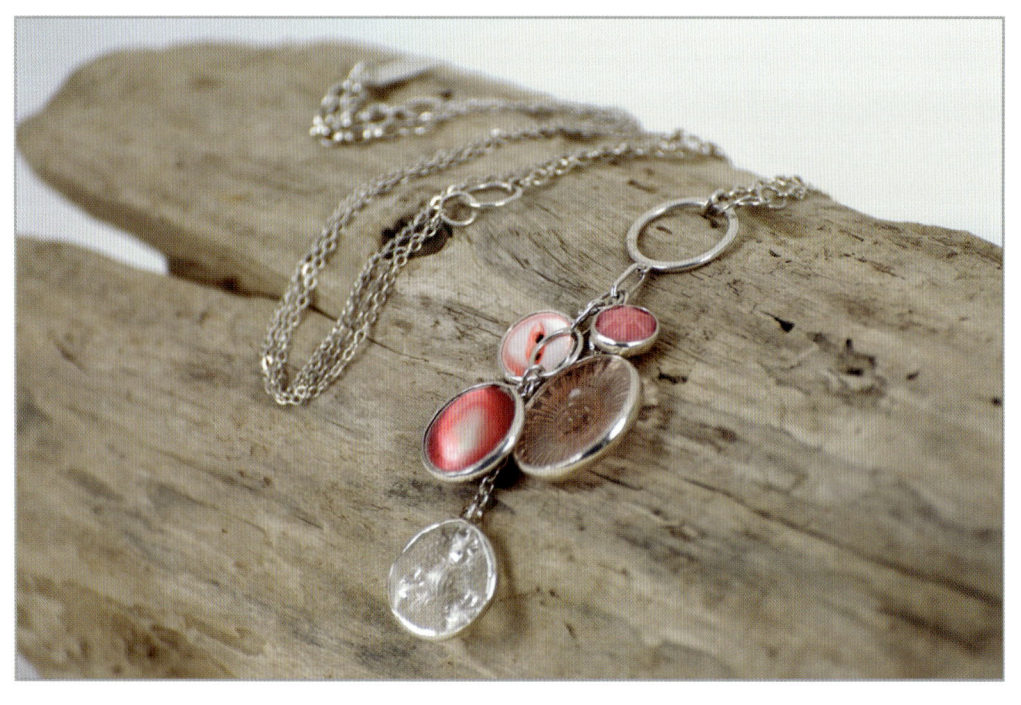

info@heatherstowell.com
www.heatherstowell.com
+44(0)1638739197

CHAPTER TEN: ABOUT THE DESIGNERS

Hannah Souter

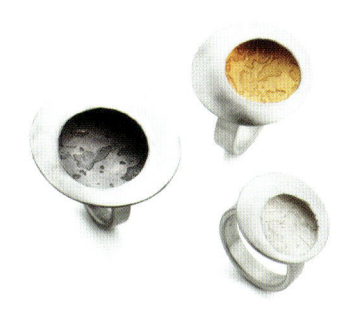

In 2002 Hannah graduated from Kent Institute of Art and Design with a first class BA (Hons) in Silversmithing, Goldsmithing and Jewellery Design. She then refined her skills with a one year post-graduate residency for jewellers and silversmiths at Bishopsland Workshops in Reading.

"Inspired by the beauty and delicate structures in the natural world I create sculptural jewellery. Working in precious metals such as silver and 18ct gold my jewellery is comprised of hand pressed and individually fabricated units combined with subtle surface textures and contrasting finishes to create unique sculptural jewellery."

Hannah's etched range (new in 2011) has proved to be in very high demand. The inner surfaces of the domed discs are etched with nitric acid to produce an interesting and tactile surface. The interior of the domes are either left with a matt silver finish, oxidized to form a dark grey interior or plated with 22ct gold.

Hannah sells her work at craft and design fairs across the country, through a selection of prestigious galleries and via her web site. Her jewellery appeals to a vast cross section of people due to her range of different sized pieces and variety of the finishes.

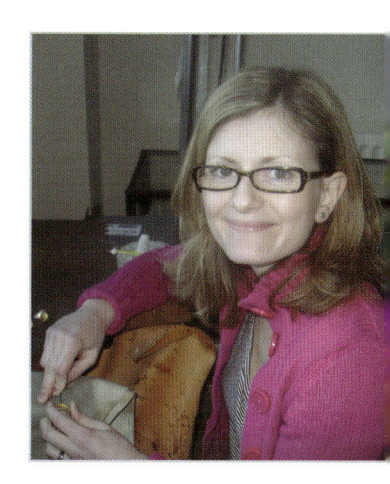

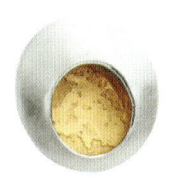

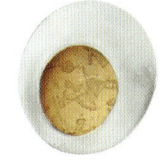

www.hannahsouter.co.uk
hannahsouter@hotmail.com
+44(0)7789910928

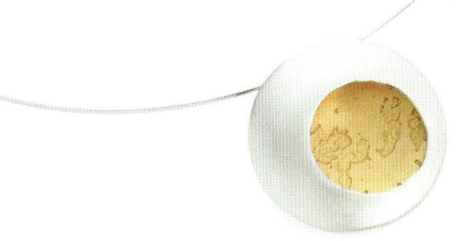

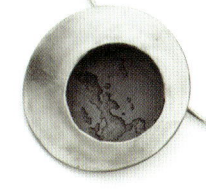

99

DOES THIS LOOK GOOD ON ME?

Emma Turpin

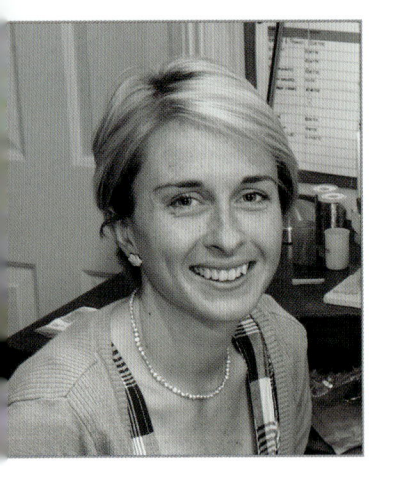

Emma is an Essex based jeweller with a passion for traditional Crafts and Craftsmanship. Emma draws inspiration from Victorian Folk life, Victorian interiors and buildings.

Emma explains *"I am continually striving to create Contemporary wearable pieces of jewellery with the essence of bringing the old with the new together."*

Emma graduated from Middlesex University in 2005, during which time she explored the beginnings of her main collection 'Maidens Garlands' which consists of handfolded fine silver rosettes, a technique developed by Emma. Her love for the bygone era influences many of her designs including her new 'Frame Collection' with its sharp lines and sculptural shapes incorporating semi precious stones. Emma works in silver, 18ct gold with elements of oxidisation and 22ct gold plating.

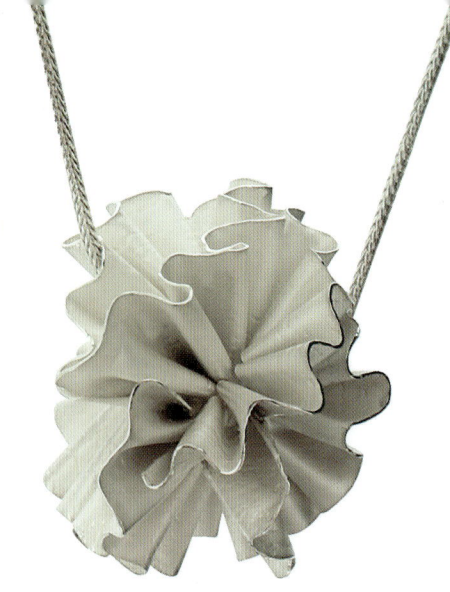

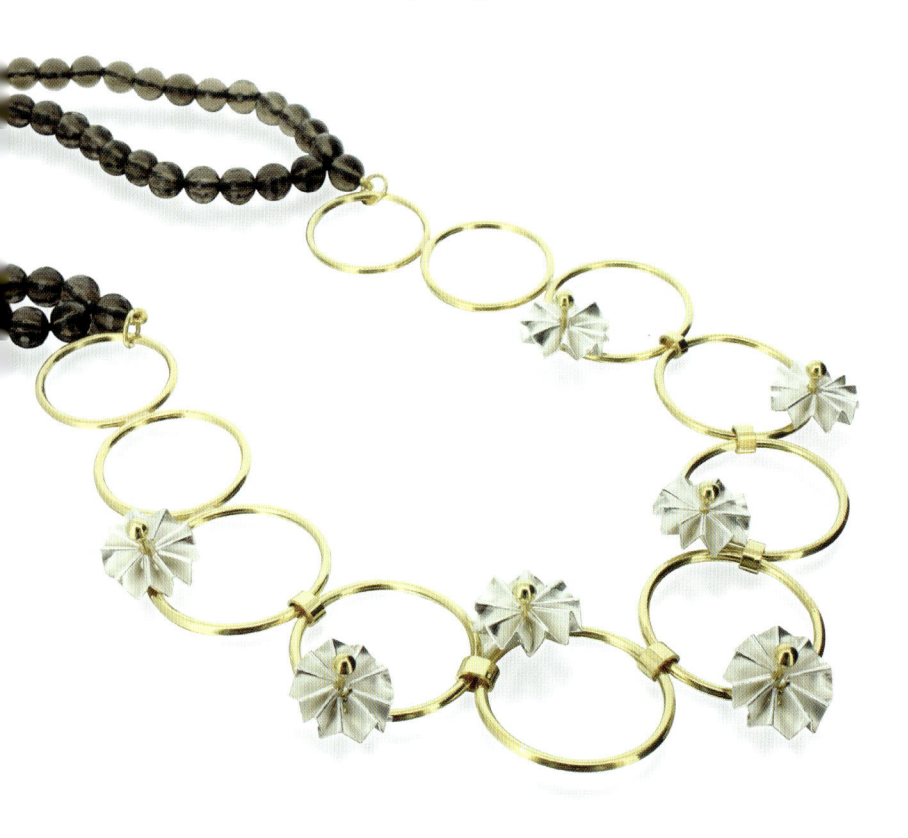

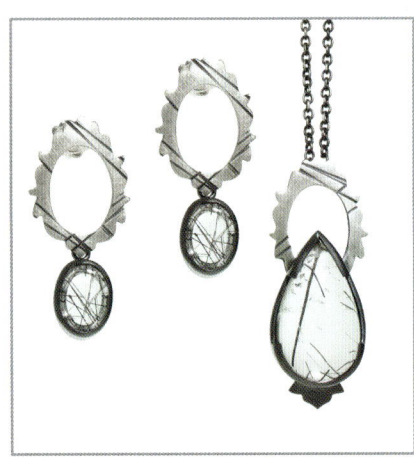

www.emmaturpin.com
info@emmaturpin.com
+44(0)7860749299

CHAPTER TEN: ABOUT THE DESIGNERS

Susanne Tweddle

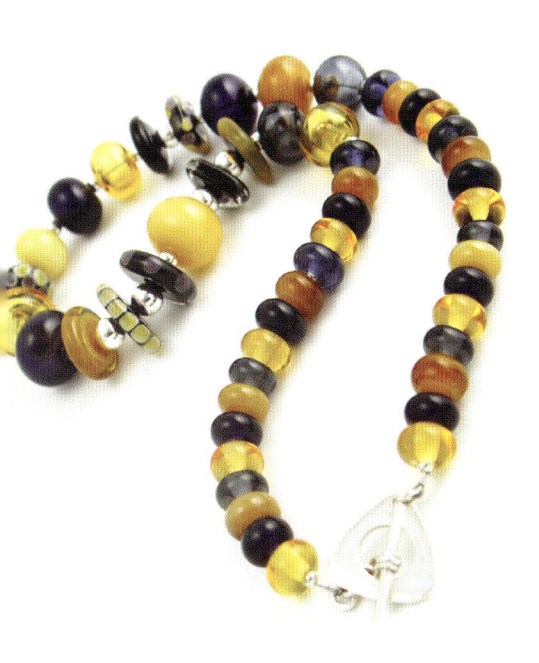

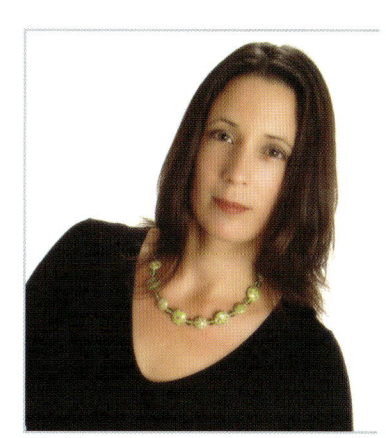

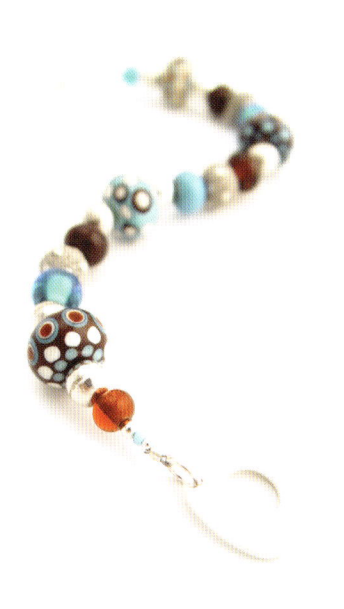

Susanne graduated in design at the University of Derbyshire in 1992, specializing in the manufacture and design of jewellery. Lampworking has enabled Susanne to inject vibrancy and colour into her work, offering contrast to silver and the other materials she uses in her designs. In April 2004 Susanne set up business as 'Susanne – Glass Beads & Jewellery Designer'.

Susanne individually makes each of the glass beads using a lampworking technique. *"I love watching each bead grow and develop,"* says Susanne, who works from a workshop at her home in County Durham. *"And I still get a real buzz opening the door of the kiln 12 hours later. It's the anticipation of what I might find."* Susanne's feel for colour - and how she contrasts this with the silver and other materials she uses - is what really sets her work apart. *"It's colour that inspires my designs. From the brightest oranges to the coolest blues, I am always experimenting with different combinations. I use mainly Venetian glass for its spectacular colour range and clarity."* Susanne adds, *"the inclusion of other techniques such as etching, fine silver, silver leaf detail and enameling in my most recent designs has added new textures and subtle colours to my beads. The techniques I use have been around for 1000s of years but my interpretation of design and colour sets my beads and jewellery apart."*

Susanne's customer base is vast and varied, the only stereotype being someone who demands individual, handmade, colourful jewellery and appreciates the skill and techniques used to manufacture it.

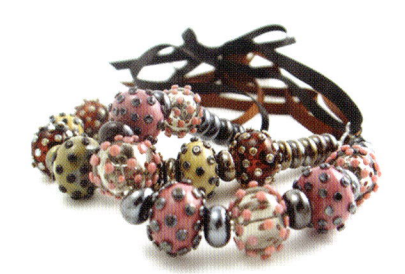

www.Susannejewellery.co.uk
Susanne@Susannejewellery.co.uk
+44(0)1833638625

101

Does This Look Good On Me?

Susan Vedadi

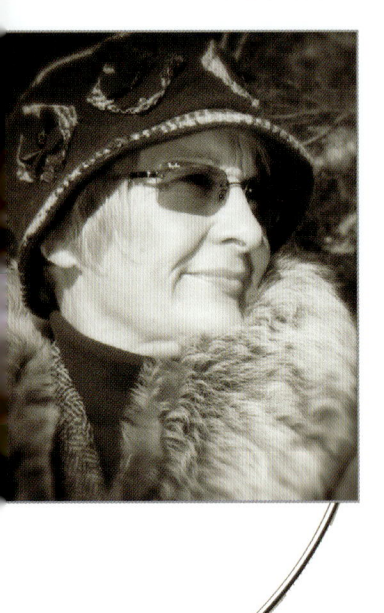

Susan works in the heart of Birmingham's jewellery quarter, where she has run her own business since the 1970s. After leaving school she spent a year as a trainee at the Herbert Art Gallery & Museum, Coventry but left to go to Birmingham and take a BA course in Three Dimensional Design specialising in jewellery. Apart from six months living in Paris she has stayed rooted in the jewellery quarter, enjoying having all of the jewellery allied trades on her doorstep.

She is a Freeman of the Goldsmiths Company and has work in the permanent collection of Birmingham City Art Gallery & Museum. Over the years she has exhibited at the Goldsmiths Fair, Art in Action, with The Designer Jewellers Group and has had work in Electrum, Roger Billcliffe Glasgow, Dazzle at the National Theatre, Centrepiece at Symphony Hall, Birmingham and many more.

Her main outlets have always been selected craft fairs where she enjoys sharing her enthusiasm for her one-off designs and the unusual and rare gemstones she uses. Working mainly in 18ct. gold her work draws its influences from her love of all periods of antique jewellery and the colour and unique qualities of gems.

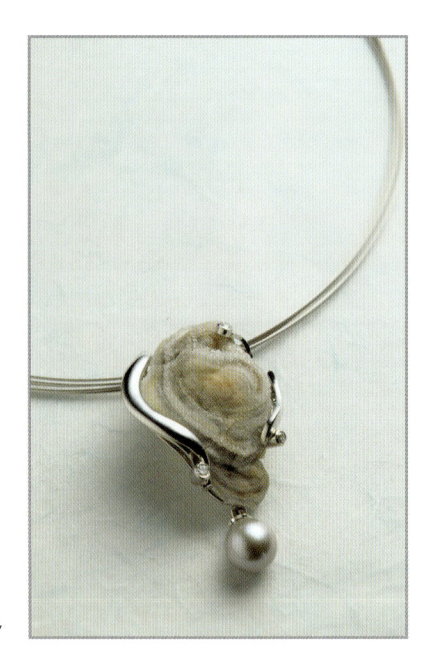

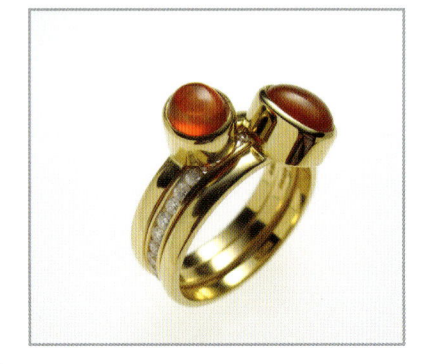

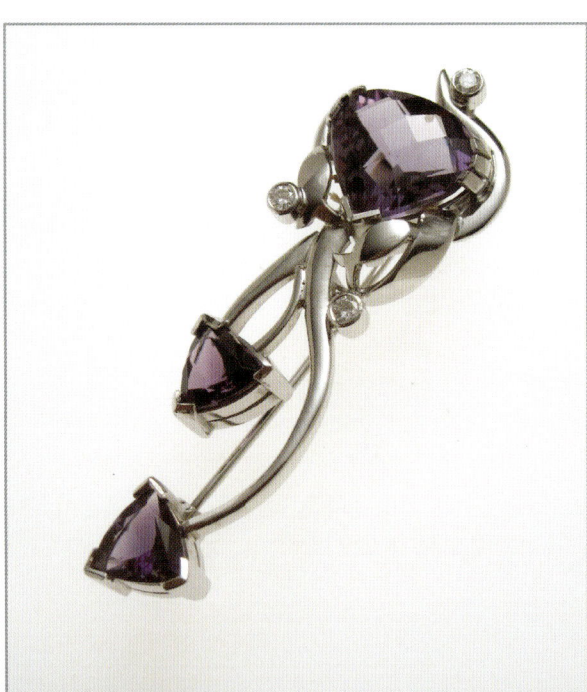

www.susanvedai.com
info@susanvedadi.com
+44(0)7768592552

102

CHAPTER TEN: ABOUT THE DESIGNERS

Liz Willis

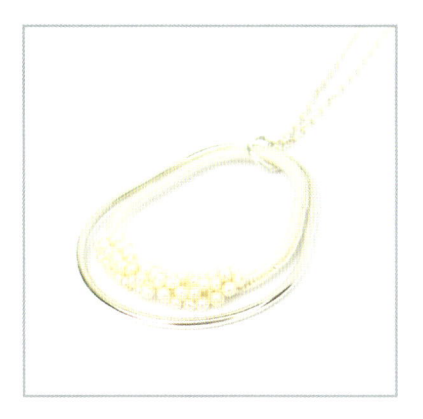

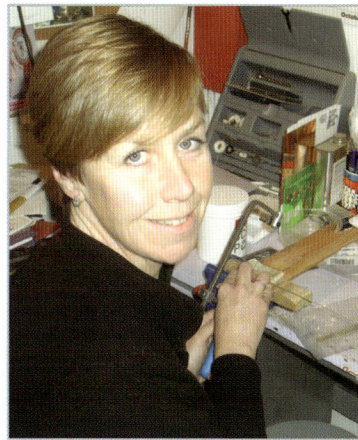

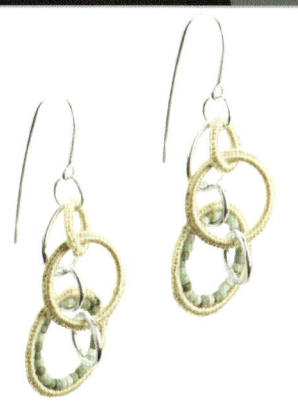

Liz graduated from the University of Hertfordshire in 2008 with a BA in Applied Arts. She is a member of the Association for Contemporary Jewellery and a licentiate member of the Society of Designer Craftsmen. She has developed her skills further with a work placement in the prestigious workshop of Ute Decker (Sept-Nov 2011).

"My work is inspired by the environments that I see around me while out running. Travelling on foot through the landscape allows us a greater appreciation of the colours, contours and textures of the world around us, and gives us the opportunity to see aspects of the environment not often noticed in the rush and chaos of day-to-day life.

Each piece evolves from an aspect of a run that catches my attention, from flat slate pebbles on a beach that slide sideways when stepped on, or a footpath disappearing down a lichen-rich tree tunnel, to being surrounded by the vibrant colours and noises of a large road race like the London Marathon.

I use silver and gold wire to form an appropriate shape for the piece, and then hand stitch over part or all of it with silk threads, occasionally using pearls or semi-precious stone or glass beads, to add the colour and texture relevant to the run I am trying to portray. Although this is a time consuming process, it does mean that I am constantly reminded of my favourite places to run whilst I work!"

"Slowness gives you eyes in your feet and can be a catalyst for the senses"
Rosie Swale Pope

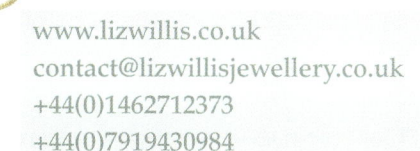

www.lizwillis.co.uk
contact@lizwillisjewellery.co.uk
+44(0)1462712373
+44(0)7919430984

103

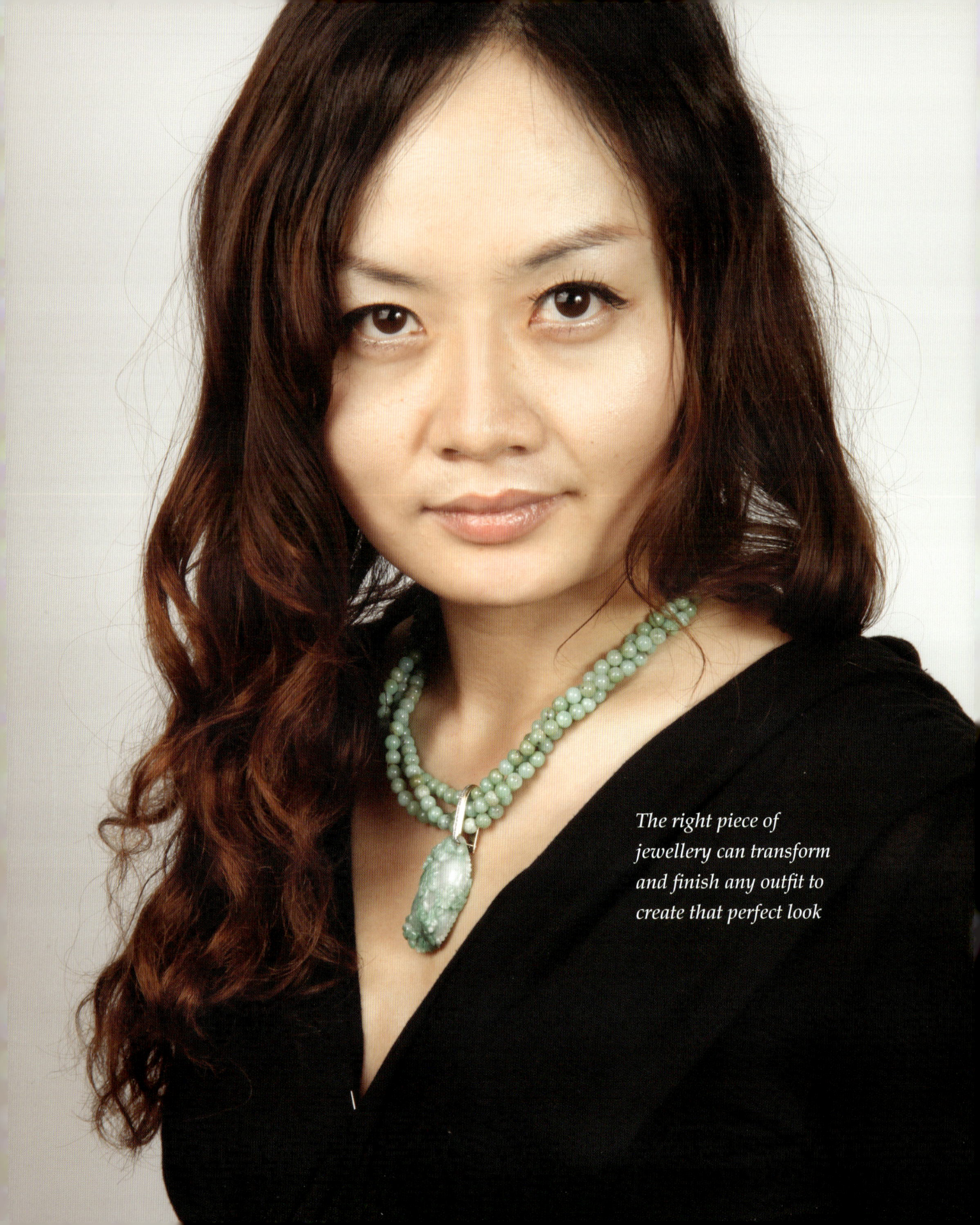

The right piece of jewellery can transform and finish any outfit to create that perfect look

Putting it all together

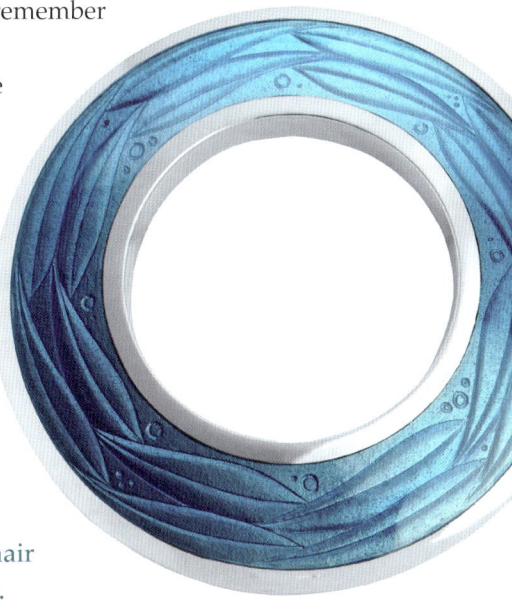

Jewellery is important. It brings an outfit together by adding those finishing touches. Jewellery can transform a day outfit into one suitable for an evening function. Jewellery can be expensive or affordable, understated or flamboyant but it always adds to your image and style; it is a window offering the viewer an insight into your personality.

When you are selecting your jewellery remember to take into account your physical characteristics, your personality and the occasion when you will be wearing it.

Consider:

- Face Shape – indicates the size, shape and type of earring and suggests an appropriate necklace type.

- Neck length and width – determines whether you will suit long, dangly earrings and short or choker style necklaces

- Colouring – the colour of your skin, hair and eye decide what colours suit you.

- Age – can determine if a style of jewellery is appropriate.

- Personality – are you a Classic, Romantic, Casual or Creative? The answer to this question can help you decide if the jewellery 'sits well with you' and can help avoid the expense of buying jewellery that you will not wear.

- Occasion – where you are going and what you are going to do when you get there is important in determining what jewellery is appropriate to wear.

There is a wealth of jewellery on the market to suit every conceivable individual and occasion. Wear it and enjoy it! Using the advice in this book, the answer to the question "Does this look good on me?" will be "Yes," always.

Recommended Reading

colour me beautiful - expert advice to help you feel confident and look great by Veronique Henderson & Pat Henshaw with colour me beautiful the image consultants.
Hamlyn 2010
ISBN978-0-600-62080-8

Colour Me Beautiful - Discover your natural beauty through colour by Carole Jackson.
Piatkus 1989
ISBN 0-86188-299-7

Always In Style - Develop your own personal image with shape and colour by Doris Pooser.
Piatkus 1987
ISBN 0-86188-699-2

Wardrobe - Develop your style and confidence by Suxie Faux with Philipa Davies.
Piatkus 1988
ISBN 0-86188-726-3

Acknowledgments

I would like to thank all of the following for their invaluable help and support, without which this book would never have come into being:

The models:
Evelyn Barber
Beverley De'Asha
Danielle Faulkner-Dunkley
Helena Holricks
Jade O'Kane
Sarah Tarry

The designer makers
Carole Allen
Lyn Antley
Daniela Dobesova
Theresa Galanides (Minimal Marzipan)
Rachel Gogerly
Simone Micallef
Shivani Patel
Heather Stowell
Hannah Souter
Emma Turpin
Susan Vedadi
Liz Willis

Others

Design and typesetting:
Jane Bigos of Clockwork Graphic Design

Photography:
Neil Ginger of Ginger Photography

Editing and publishing:
Sarah Williams of The Book Consultancy and The Wordsmith Press

And finally thank you to my husband Bruce, children Danielle and Michael and mother Christine for their love, support and understanding.

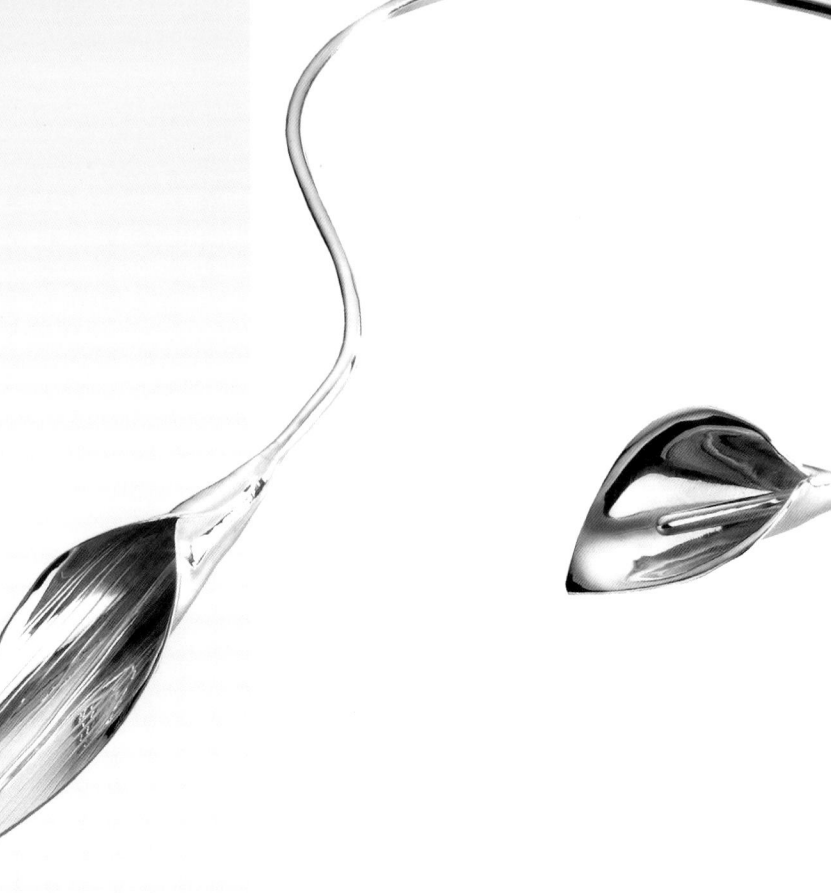